Triple Coronary Bypass

A Cardiologist Tells about His and How to Prevent Yours

Clifford G. Gaddy, M.D.

Mercer University Press

ISBN 0-86554-447-6 MUP/P109

Triple Coronary Bypass.
A Cardiologist Tells about His and How to Prevent Yours.

Mercer University Press, Macon, Georgia 31207 USA

Printed in the United States of America

The paper used in this publication meets
the minumum requirements of American National Standard
for Information Sciences—Permanence of Paper
for Printed Library Materials, ANSI Z39.48–1984.

Library of Congress Cataloging-in-Publication Data

Gaddy, Clifford G. (Clifford Garland), 1924– .
Triple coronary bypass : a cardiologist tells about his
and how to prevent yours / Clifford G. Gaddy.
xi+104pp. 6x9" (15x23cm.).
ISBN 0-86554-447-6 (alk. paper).
1. Coronary artery bypass—popular works.
2. Coronary heart disease—Prevention.
3. Gaddy, Clifford G. (Clifford Garland), 1924– —Health.
I. Title.
[DNLM: 1. Gaddy, Clifford G. (Clifford Garland), 1924– .
2. Coronary Artery Bypass—personal narratives.
3. Coronary Disease—prevention & control. WG 113 G123t 1994]
RD 598.35.C67G33 1994
617.4'12—dc20
DNLM/CLC
for Library of Congress 94-17535
CIP

Table of Contents

List of Illustrations

Preface

In October 1992, I had coronary bypass surgery. After I arrived home following surgery, I began jotting down some notes about the events leading up to my chest pain and the resulting measures taken. I had in mind primarily information that might be of interest to myself and to my family in the years ahead.

Several aspects of my experiences struck me. For one thing, a sixty-eight-year-old physician having a heart attack while making a high-wire rope walk is an unusual event. For another, an experienced cardiologist ought to have recognized my preceding chest pains as being due to heart disease. I might have taken steps to deal with stress factors which contributed to the development of my coronary heart disease. Also, a more careful prior evaluation of my family medical history would have been in order.

My family and friends encouraged me in this journal. When I casually mentioned my project to Dr. Robert Jones, my surgeon, at my six weeks' checkup back at Duke Medical Center, he reacted with enthusiasm, encouraging me to develop it for publication. He thought it would be helpful for those with heart problems, especially those anticipating surgery.

My reactions to my experience undoubtedly were different from those of anyone else. I have tried to express them in an honest fashion, hoping that in some way they may prove helpful to others who are anticipating similar procedures. My treatment was not necessarily the ideal one for every patient. What I did in my post-surgical personal management will not reflect what every patient should do for himself. First, last, and in-between, a patient should follow the advice of his own physician.

I address the risk factors responsible for producing cholesterol defects in the coronary arteries, and point out how to deal with these problems. The use of medications in the management of cholesterol and associated heart disease is touched on only briefly, because I feel this is a decision that should be made between the patient and his or her own physician.

With this book I hope to improve understanding of the process of coronary bypass surgery. Equally important, I hope it will lead to precautions that may prevent the consequences I have suffered.

June 1993 *Clifford G. Gaddy, M.D.*

Acknowledgments

Under circumstances as complex as I have encountered, it is difficult to acknowledge all of those who were so helpful.

There were those who managed my illness, starting with the onset of chest pain while at our family retreat. I am indebted to Dr. Thomas Farmer and the Emergency Room staff at Transylvania County Hospital in Brevard, North Carolina, for their immediate care.

Dr. Ruffin Benton and the Coronary Care nurses treated me with the utmost care and consideration. I received the most careful attention possible.

I will always be grateful to Dr. Robert Califf for arranging my transfer to the Duke Medical Center by an outstanding Life Flight crew.

Dr. Robert Peter and his catheterization team demonstrated consummate knowledge and skill in performing my angiograms.

Dr. Robert Jones, my cardiac surgeon, and his magnificent support group did a remarkable job with bypass surgery. No patient could have been more fortunate in the care that I received.

My wife Nez gave me the greatest possible support throughout, from the high-wire rope walk where it all started to my rehabilitation. I can't imagine what it might have been like to have been without her support every step of the way.

The preparation of a manuscript is a difficult task. I had almost no experience in typing or using a computer for word processing. Foremost, I have to credit my son Steve for his help with the computer. I jokingly credit him with keeping me from having another heart attack during the preparation of the manuscript. Pam Reese and Betty Parrish of Medical Word Processing, and Beryl Clifton and Doris Hall of my office secretarial staff have been very helpful.

Martha and Rodney Beals and Dot Adams are among many who have helped me with editing and proofreading. Stanley Hall, M.D., of Medical College of Virginia, has been very helpful in making suggestions. Dr. Robert Whalen and Dr. Robert Jones checked the manuscript for accuracy regarding the medical data and procedures. Help came from many others too numerous to name. I thank my literary agent John White and my publisher, Dr. Cecil P. Staton, Jr. They have provided outstanding professional help. Joe Gaddy, my oldest grandson, has helped with the illustrations.

Again, I must acknowledge the tolerance and help Nez has provided during the preparation of the manuscript.

Clifford G. Gaddy, M.D.

Dedication

I dedicate this book to my family.

Since I first met Nez
my life has been so very fulfilling
because of her devotion to me
and to the goals I have set for my life.

I am so fortunate to have a family that has provided me
so much pleasure and satisfaction.
Each of our six children and their spouses,
in their own way,
has given me a sense of pride about their achievements.
Our relationships have always been more
than the usual parent-child relationship.
I will always have a feeling of security as long as I have them.
They are my best friends and I think the feeling is mutual.

To be loved is wonderful!
To also be liked is great!

A Family Retreat in the Mountains

When my wife Inez—she prefers Nez—and I set out for the mountains of North Carolina on Friday, October 9, 1992, I had no idea that the events of the next seven days would change our lives forever.

It is a tradition for our family to get together about twice each year. Our immediate family consists of twenty-six members. It is easy to keep up with because there are six children, their six spouses, six grandsons and six granddaughters. Steve, our second son, and his wife Beth had grown quite fond of Eagle's Nest Camp, near Brevard, North Carolina. Steve had arranged for us to meet at the camp on Friday for a three-day weekend. All were able to attend except Cliff, our oldest son, and his family of four, who were about nine hours away in Maryland, and Bobby, our fourth son, and his wife Evelyn, who live in Gloucester, Virginia, about eight hours from the camp.

Nez and I arrived early and were met by Rich Campbell, director of the camp for our weekend. He showed us to our eating and sleeping quarters. We had a chance to hike around and explore the area before anyone else arrived.

Betty, our oldest daughter, arrived early, bringing four-year-old Carolyn and two-year-old Emma. Betty's husband Bill was to arrive later. Betty, a pediatrician in Raleigh, immediately challenged me to a game of tennis. Smart girl! She knew I had not played tennis in more than a decade. Because of an injury to my neck three or four decades ago, serving the ball caused pain in my neck, chest, and arms. Yet I agreed, even to the use of Carolyn's racket. I knew I would want excuses and, needless to say, I didn't win a game. I had neck and chest pains, just as I had anticipated, but they disappeared as soon as play was over. For several years I have said that I would not know when or if I developed chest pain on exertion (called angina pectoris) due to heart trouble, because the old injury had caused arthritis of my neck and the activities that would aggravate my neck pain could also cause angina.

Gary, a Ph.D. in Communications Research from the University of North Carolina, arrived from Chapel Hill with his wife Becky and their two boys, Joe and Matt.

Steve, who works as an Investment Management Consultant, and his wife Beth were our host and hostess of a sort, since they alone were familiar with Camp Eagle's Nest. Their daughters Heather, Erin, and Anne Marie had each attended summer camp there for several years.

We missed our evening orientation session because of the late arrival of Janet, our second daughter, and her family. Janet's husband Robi had been detained at school, counseling a student with emotional problems. They brought their three boys, John, Jeremy, and Jason.

On Saturday morning, we were offered a choice of canoeing or rock climbing. The hiking and climbing instructors led their group off to the mountains. I couldn't wait to join the group going to shoot the white water rapids on the Green River. I had no previous experience with white water, but had the good fortune to be teamed with Heather, who has canoed before at camp. After brief instructions on the lake at camp, we headed out to the river, twenty miles off. Only Bill, a grandson of the late coach Bill Murray of Duke University, who prides himself on being a good all-round athlete and Janet, tipped over their canoe in the lake during practice exercises. Naturally, we did not let them forget this.

To reach our starting point, we traveled some four or five miles up a mountain trail where we put our canoes into the river. Before taking off in our canoes, we devoured a high-energy snack of sandwiches and fruit.

We skimmed about four miles downstream through the rapids, which were rated only grade one and two, the easiest degrees. Nevertheless, we bounced off a fair number of rocks and reversed our course several times. Occasionally, we had to hold up and wait for a canoe that had tipped over. Heather and I were the only ones who arrived dry.

During vigorous paddling, I felt the usual pains in my neck, chest and between my shoulder blades, just as I had with tennis. On reaching the eddies, where rest was possible, the discomfort always subsided. I hoped this was only my old neck arthritis. I did ask myself, "Is this angina?" but dismissed the question because white-water canoeing was a delightful experience that I did not want to cut short and everyone was having a wonderful time.

That evening we invited Jack and Gwen Dickerson, old friends who lived nearby, over for the evening meal. Jack is a physician recently retired from thirty-five years of surgery in Waynesville, North Carolina. I considered telling Jack about my chest pains but I decided against it. He would have insisted on my having it checked right away, and I didn't want anything to interfere with our family weekend. I concluded that the chest pain could wait. I did promise myself to have it checked out on returning home.

The Original Injury

Neck and arm pains have been a problem for me for more than thirty years. It began when our oldest son Clifford Jr. was nine or ten years old. We were engaged in a bit of horseplay. I was holding him over my head. When I thought he would fall onto the hardwood floor, I allowed him to fall on top of my head. I suffered a compression of the vertebral discs in my neck, causing transient numbness and tingling with loss of use of my arms, which, momentarily, I could not move. Breathing was difficult. For an instant I thought I was going to be paralyzed.

For many months I wore a cervical collar for neck support. I spent many nights in traction. Nez massaged my neck and applied hot packs and electric pads. This went on, not for weeks or months, but for years. With continued physical therapy, including ultrasound, hot packs, traction, and whirlpool, both at the Danville Memorial Hospital Physical Therapy Department, and at home, I gradually improved, but the discomfort never fully disappeared.

For reasons that are not clear to me, about ten years ago my neck pain significantly worsened. After seeing internists, neurologists, chiropractors, acupuncturists, and a faith healer who came to see me, I received no significant relief. I was admitted twice to my alma mater, Bowman Gray School of Medicine in Winston-Salem, North Carolina. I was evaluated by Dr. Michael McWhorter and Dr. James Toole, who on both occasions felt that surgery on my neck would not be justified. I had many X-rays, computerized tomography (CT; or computed axial tomography, CAT) scans and magnetic resonance imaging (MRI), as well as nerve conduction studies. The pain was never severe, but there was a persistent discomfort, particularly interfering with my rest at night. I arranged with my colleagues at the office to do part-time work. At the hospital I was granted a status known as Courtesy Hospital Staff Physician. This status exempted me from emergency calls and hospital work.

I was given rotating neck exercises. While these were uncomfortable, I do feel that I realized long-term benefits. I gave up tennis but continued other activities, including golf.

By the time I was twenty-nine Nez and I had four sons. The boys and I sort of grew up together. It was fun. It gave me a chance to have the electric train that I never had as a child, and to help build a go-cart. I didn't take up golf until I was forty-five, although I knew I would like the game. I had seen too many golf orphans, and besides, I was having too much fun being one of the boys. They expected me to do whatever they did, and so did I. This probably helps explain my stubborn insistence on making the high-wire rope walk.

The Rope Walk

Sunday was our third and last day at Camp Eagle's Nest. After we sang our morning blessing led by our granddaughter Anne Marie, and had breakfast, we made our way to the high-wire rope-walk course. This would be the real highlight of our weekend. Our counselors gave us detailed instructions on how to put on our climbing gear and helmets. When we attached and carefully checked our safety belts, we called, "On Belay"—which means "My rope is secured"—to the instructor in charge. This was to assure our safety in the event of a fall.

The course was divided into three parts. The first was a semivertical climb to a point about thirty feet above the ground. Here the safety rope was detached, passed around the tree and reattached to the belt. Again each one of us called "On Belay" to the instructor before beginning the first wire walk. You were able to stabilize yourself with an overhead horizontal cable during the first walk, and this was not so difficult.

The second portion of the wire walk became much more difficult, in that you had only the assistance of a single rope attached to the tree from which you began to use as leverage to reach the next destination about forty feet away. The final leg was that of walking, unassisted, a twelve inch diameter pole at a height of thirty feet. Some, especially Gary, found this the most difficult part. For descent, you took a backward free fall, secured only by the safety rope controlled by one of our counselors, who lowered us to the ground.

Our most skilled climbers, Matt, Joe, and Erin, were first to climb. They were cheered on by the rest of the group as they reached each point toward their destination. As the group got older, and in general somewhat heavier, the progress became tougher.

Finally, the eldest of the group opted to take his turn. Nez did not like the idea, being concerned that I might aggravate my neck pains, which was all she knew of my symptoms. I did well until the second-stage wire walk, when I was aided only by the heavy-duty fabric rope. I had envisioned the challenge of the course as being primarily one of psychologically adapting to heights. However, I soon found that it was physically very strenuous. There was a great deal of isometric contraction of the muscles of the arms and legs, which are specifically to be avoided by heart patients. I developed neck and chest pains, even worse than I had at tennis or paddling the white water rapids.

I heard lots of encouragement from the kids watching. "You can do it, Dad! Hang in there!" they called. No one suggested that I give up the effort. Nez later reported that she thought I looked pale and sweaty. She wanted me to give up the course and be let down to the ground by the safety rope. But she has never played the role of an overprotective wife and mother. She took little Emma and walked away from the scene. I read this accurately as an indication of her concern. If only in consideration of Nez's feeling, I should have asked that the walk be cut short and had myself lowered to the ground.

Even after pausing about midway through the course, the pains did not subside. I could not be sure if my sweating was due to pain or exertion. I knew that the course was intended for teenagers and young adults, but I did not want to give up, so I completed the walk to the applause of my children and grandchildren.

I was confident while on the high wire that I was having heart pain. I only hoped that it would subside. I was anxious not to cast a spell over what had been such a great weekend. In my medicine kit, I always carried nitroglycerin, a medication commonly used for angina pectoris. I had never suspected that I would need it for myself, but kept it available should anyone in my presence ever have a bout of suspected angina. I put two of the nitroglycerin tablets under my tongue at about five-minute intervals. No relief. My concern increased, but I tried to conceal it.

After I had been on the ground for ten minutes or so, I confessed my chest pain to Nez. She only commented, "I knew you were foolish to be up there." I told her that I must have it evaluated.

Is This Angina Pectoris?

My fear was of "angina pectoris," a term that technically means "pain in the chest," but has come to designate chest pain associated with inadequate circulation to the heart. I have been describing it to patients for more than forty years. In most instances there is diminished circulation to the heart muscle because of narrowing of the coronary arteries. Characteristically, the pain comes on when the heart is put under strain, such as during exercise, or emotional stress. It tends to subside with rest or alleviation of the stressful circumstance. The discomfort usually disappears with allowing one or two tablets of a nitrate medication called nitroglycerin, to dissolve underneath the tongue.

We now know that angina can sometimes be provoked by a spasm of the coronary arteries, which may occur during stress, and is observed even in very young people after the use of cocaine. Most frequently, the hurting is felt in the front of the chest behind the breast bone and may radiate into the shoulders or arms, more often on the left side. It is often described as a feeling of weight or heaviness on the chest. A common expression is, "It feels like a ton of bricks on my chest." The discomfort is often vague, and may be considered indigestion rather than heart disease. Occasionally, it may also be felt as pain in the jaws, or between the shoulder blades in the back of the chest. On one occasion I treated an elderly man admitted to the hospital with pain only in his wrists. He had no chest pain, but his electrocardiogram confirmed an acute heart attack.

There is a somewhat unusual variation of angina that comes on at rest and is defined by a different type of change in the electrocardiogram from what we ordinarily see during angina associated with exertion. I had the good fortune of hearing Dr. Myron Prinzmetal's original presentation regarding this type of angina in 1955 at the American College of Physicians meeting in Chicago. It has subsequently been known as Prinzmetal's angina. Here coronary artery disease is usually present, but the pain seems to be secondary to the spasm of the coronary artery.

Although my chest pain was brought on by exertion, it was not typical angina for three reasons. (1) My pain was in my back between my shoulder blades, rather than in front. It did not extend into my arms. (2) The pain did not subside with rest. Characteristically, with rest the demand for blood circulation to the heart is diminished and the pain subsides. (3) It did not respond to tablets of nitroglycerin placed under my tongue.

Heart pain that persists in the presence of rest and nitroglycerin is referred to as "pre-infarction angina." This is a circumstance that is most likely to lead to a heart attack with a blood clot, producing damage to the heart muscle, which we refer to as "myocardial infarction."

Previous Concerns about My Chest Pains

I had become more concerned about my chest discomfort in the preceding eighteen to twenty-four months. I had not let it interfere with my usual activity. I continued to move heavy landscape timbers and stones, and use a moderately heavy chainsaw. I hoped the exercise would improve the arthritic stiffness in my neck. Nez argued that it would make it worse. I could not be sure. It did aggravate it at the time, but I hoped that the long-range effect might be good.

I have had four or five exercise stress tests on a treadmill over the past several years, usually without my feeling a specific need for one. I have been asked in the past how often I have a treadmill test done. I have been known to reply, "If the treadmill equipment needs testing I will volunteer."

My last treadmill study was done about eighteen months ago because I felt I might need one. I did what is called the Bruce protocol, twelve minutes of progressively more strenuous exercise. My cardiologist regarded the tracing as borderline, because of changes suggesting inadequate circulation at maximum exercise. Additionally, I grew worried about the hurting in the back of my chest between my shoulder blades during the Bruce. It was quite severe and disappeared as soon as I stepped off the treadmill. Yet, as long as I could carry one end of a railroad tie and be less short of breath than my thirty-year-old helper, I could not believe that it was anything serious.

As a cardiologist, I should have been more aware of the potential seriousness of any chest pain brought on by exertion, even in the presence of another potential cause. This is one message that I hope every reader will take to heart.

To Transylvania County Hospital

As we left Eagle's Nest I was distressed by the signs of anxiety in the children's faces. I continued to conceal my fear for the sake of the grandchildren, some of whom were not aware of my chest pain.

Nez drove the station wagon. I put my seat in the reclining position to try to relax. I observed that the degree of pain neither increased nor diminished.

I considered having Nez drive us directly to Asheville, North Carolina, some forty-five miles from the camp, for initial treatment. However, I recognized that if I *had* sustained a heart attack with a blood clot, it was important that treatment by thrombolysis (blood clot dissolvers) be started as early as possible. This has been a key advance in treatment for coronary blood clots. The earlier treatment is begun, the more effectively one can prevent damage to the heart. It is critical that treatment be administered during the first six hours after onset, although benefits can be gained up to twelve hours.

Nez and I discussed this, but elected to go to Brevard to the emergency room at the Transylvania County Hospital, that was only about three miles away. It seemed like a very long three miles.

I fully expected to find evidence of heart damage on arrival at the emergency room, and I was trying to decide on the next move. I knew Nez would agree to any reasonable choice I would make.

As soon as we arrived in front of the emergency room entrance, we were greeted by a member of the emergency room staff, who quickly took me by wheelchair to the emergency unit. I was checked by an efficient nurse who reported that my vital signs, that is, my pulse, blood pressure, and respiration, were all normal. I was promptly hooked up to a monitor that recorded my continuous electrocardiogram (EKG). The electrocardiographic unit was a modern piece of equipment that recorded each beat on an oscillograph screen, similar to a small television screen. It had the capability of

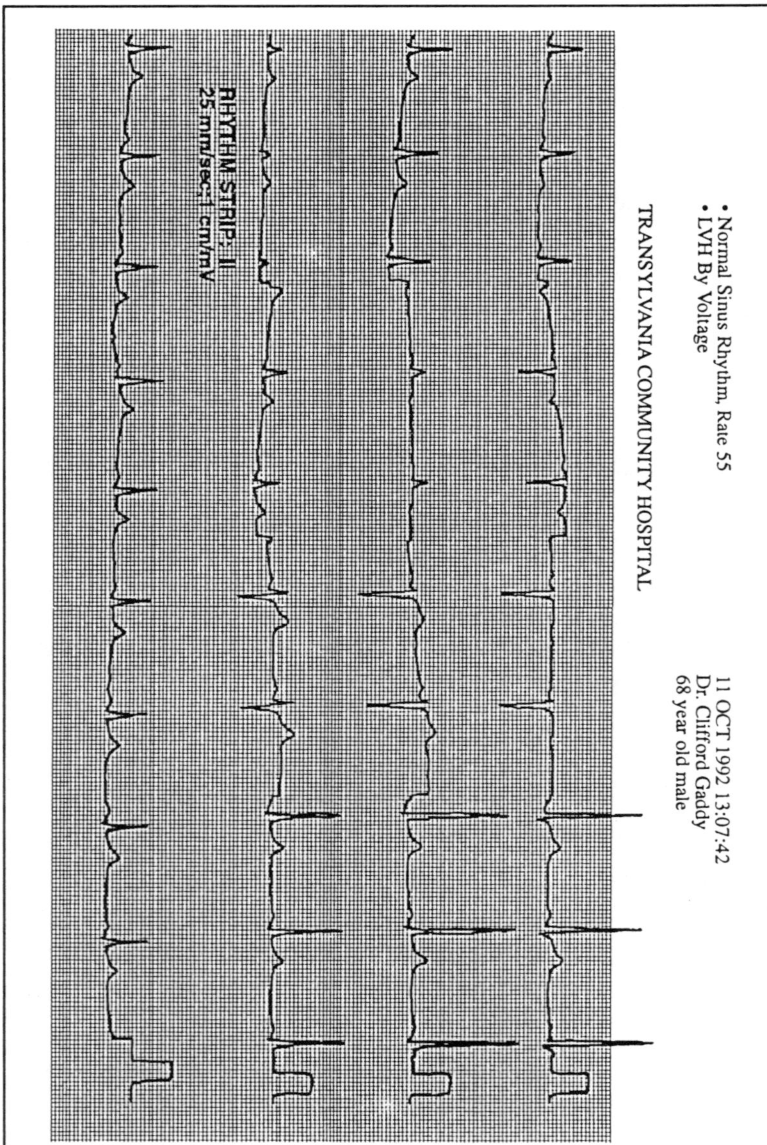

Figure 1. *Author's EKG on admission showing no change from previous tracings.*

automatically writing on electrocardiographic paper any variation from normal. This made a permanent record for the nurses and physicians to observe at the time as well as for subsequent review.

I was first checked by a physician's assistant, who observed my electrocardiogram and then handed it to me. The tracing is seen in figure 1. I agreed that the electrocardiogram was normal, unchanged from ones I have had in the past. This, of course, was reassuring to me. Nevertheless, my chest discomfort continued. What I thought I might see was an electrocardiogram with the appearance of the tracing shown in figure 2. The ST segments, that part of the EKG complex that is encircled, represent an acute blood clot producing damage to the heart muscle. Figure 2 represents an actual tracing from my files; the patient did not survive. One of my early electrocar-

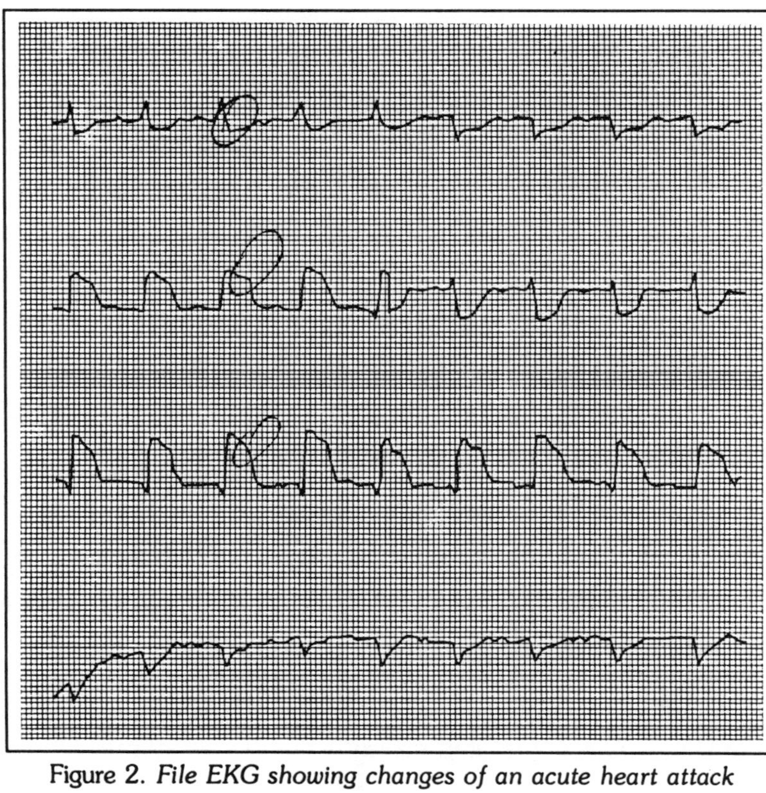

Figure 2. *File EKG showing changes of an acute heart attack with the "tombstone pattern."*

diography instructors noted the resemblance of this part of the electrocardiogram to a tombstone, an ironic indication of how serious the outlook was when such changes were noted.

By this time I had been given three additional tablets of nitroglycerin under my tongue, but there was no diminution of my chest pain. I ought to say, by the way, that my pain was never agonizing, not the heavy, crushing pain that patients often describe during an acute attack.

Fluids were being given through a vein in my arm, and a solution of nitroglycerin was being administered. The physician's assistant reported to me that he was going to place a request for the medical doctor on call for the emergency unit. Very shortly, Dr. Thomas W. Farmer arrived. I reviewed my symptoms with him and told him that the hurting had persisted since I had begun the high-wire rope walk. He suggested medication for my pain. Since the nitroglycerin had proven ineffective, I was ready for relief. He asked that the nurse prepare a dose of morphine, which is commonly used for pain in heart attacks. So far as I knew, I had never taken a dose of morphine, but many years ago I had taken Demerol for pain induced by a small kidney stone. I suggested Demerol might be preferable, not wishing to risk nausea or another side effect of morphine. A very small dose of Demerol (twenty-five milligrams) was administered and my chest pain was completely alleviated in a few minutes.

They drew blood for heart enzymes studies. The enzyme studies are quite sensitive for determining whether or not heart injury has been sustained, generally even more sensitive than the electrocardiogram. The enzymes tested are the creatinine phosphokinase (CPK) enzymes elaborated into the blood in response to any muscle injury. We anticipated that my total muscle enzymes would be elevated because of my vigorous exercise at tennis, canoeing, and rope walking during the previous three-day period, but the fraction called CPK-MB originates from the heart muscle and is characteristically elevated with heart muscle damage, such as would occur with a blood clot. The study was completed promptly and I was told that the value was fifteen units (normal would be fourteen units or less). The total

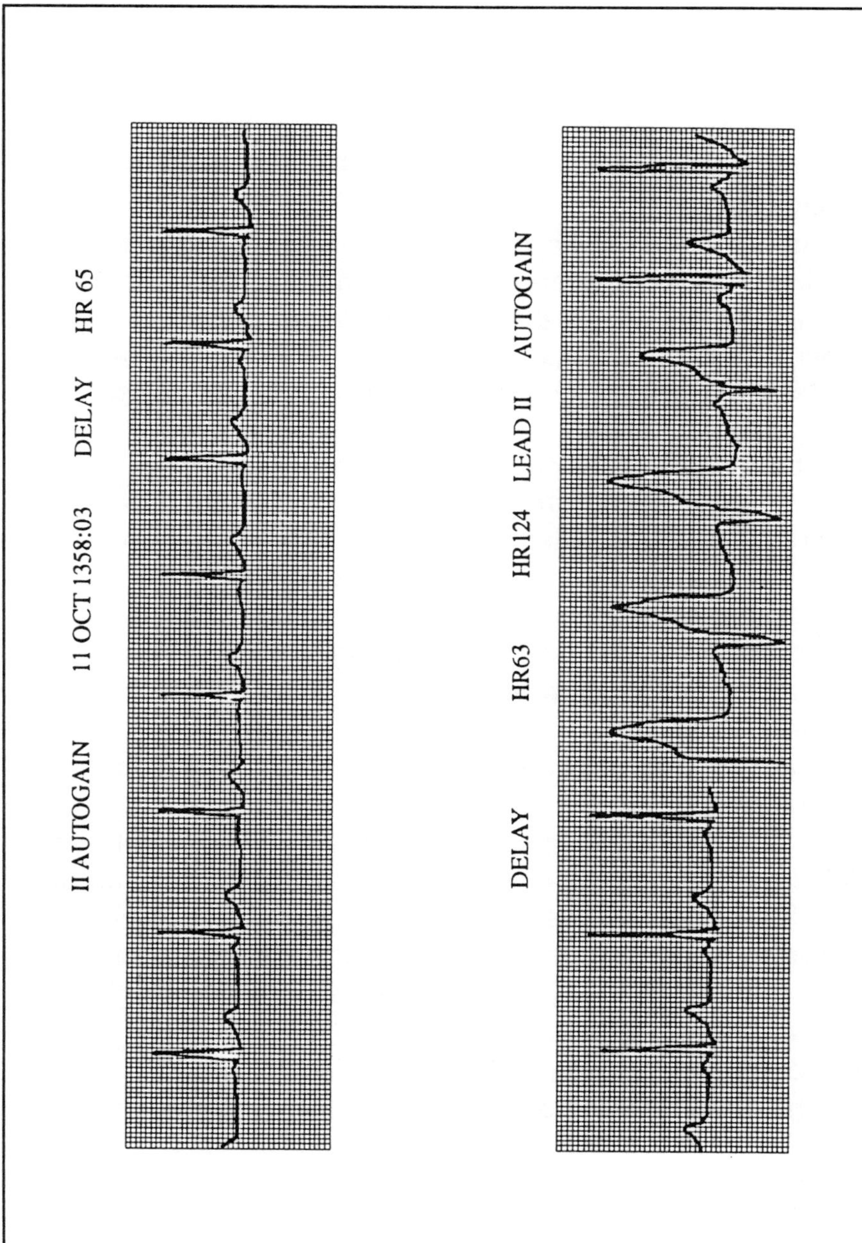

Figure 3. *Author's EKG strip taken in emergency room showing idioventricular rhythm, a sign of potential disaster. The strips are continuous.*

CPK enzymes originating from skeletal muscles were 154 units as a result of vigorous exercise (normal is less than 110 units).

In spite of the normal electrocardiogram and the favorable enzyme test, there was little doubt in my mind that my chest pain originated from my heart. It took no persuasion to keep me in the hospital for observation.

As I observed the heart monitor in the emergency room, I saw one brief episode of ventricular rhythm. See figure 3. This is a form of heartbeat that originates from an area in the ventricle of the heart, rather than in the normal upper chamber (atrium of the heart), and creates a wide complex on the EKG. When this type of beat occurs at a rapid rate, it is known as ventricular tachycardia. If not appropriately treated, this condition may lead to ventricular fibrillation, a form of fatal cardiac arrest. This is demonstrated in figure 4, which was taken from the same patient file as seen in figure 2, a case of ventricular tachycardia that did unfortunately lead to a fatal cardiac arrest.

I had observed this development on many occasions in the coronary care unit in our hospital on my patients. This time my reaction was not so detached. I said, "Oh God, is this tracing coming from my heart? This could be fatal!"

Emotions differ significantly when you are the patient rather than the doctor!

This tracing made me realize that I could at any moment require CPR (cardiopulmonary resuscitation) by the nurses and emergency medical technicians. This would entail external heart massage, and ventilation by inserting a tube in my windpipe. This would be followed by an electrical stimulus (shock) to the heart called cardioversion. As often as I have had to carry out this procedure on others, I had not before considered that this might be required for me.

The greatest feeling of anxiety that I felt up to this point came when I realized that an episode of the abnormal ventricular rhythm I had just observed might well have taken place while I was on the high wire. If it had, I would have fallen from the wire and dangled by the safety rope, while being lowered to the ground. I would have received resuscitation by individuals perhaps less well-trained in giving external

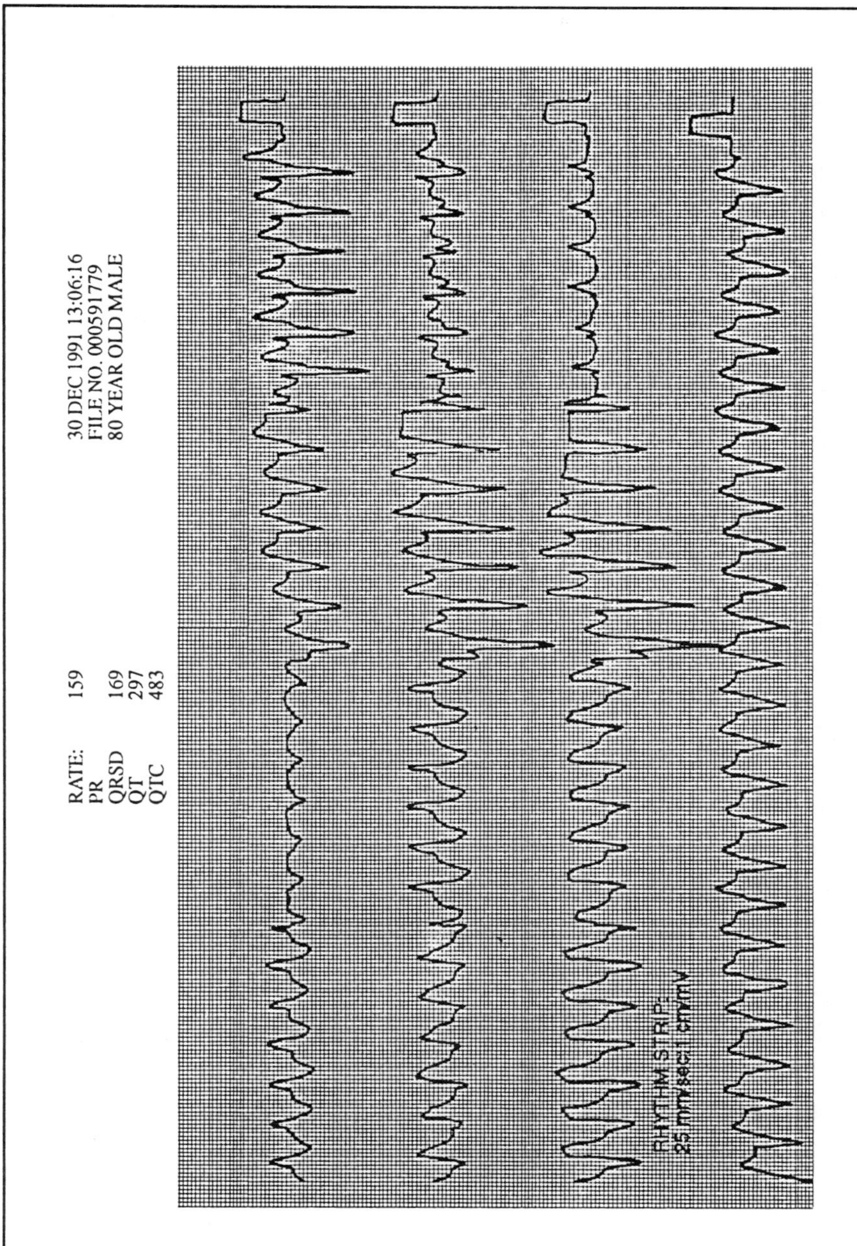

Figure 4. *File EKG taken from a patient with ventricular tachycardia, which proved fatal. (Same patient as in figure 2, above.)*

heart massage. Pulmonary resuscitation would have been merely mouth to mouth, since a tube for insertion into the wind pipe was not at hand. The lack of a ventilation bag (Ambu-bag) would have made ventilation very inefficient. A life-saving unit could not have quickly reached the camp site. The chances for a successful resuscitation would have been very poor.

These speculations are not all that cause me to shudder. I can not avoid thinking of the psychological trauma that would have resulted had this taken place in the presence of Nez, our four children and their spouses, and nine grandchildren aged two to fifteen years. In the emergency room or coronary care unit we spare the family this traumatic experience by having them wait in an adjoining room. I think I have felt as much anxiety over the possibility of my family witnessing a resuscitation as I have over a long-shot resuscitation attempt. The former would have been a lifelong anguished memory for my family. I will never forget to praise God that this did not happen.

Nez was in the admitting office giving information and did not witness the ventricular irregularity. I was glad she was not on hand because I had just reported to her that my resting electrocardiogram was normal.

Our children all checked on me in the emergency room before leaving Brevard. Each volunteered to stay with me, but I did not feel it necessary. I told them I was confident that a transfer would be in order. Each urged me to arrange for additional studies to be done closer home.

I was served a light dinner tray, which I enjoyed. No matter the state of my health, I am sure appetite will be the last life sign to go.

Nez remained with me. Characteristically, she showed no outward signs of anxiety, and her calm demeanor reassured me. I could never receive greater support. After it appeared that I had quieted down for the night, the hospital staff helped locate a motel room near the hospital. She stroked my forehead and gave me a loving, goodnight kiss.

As she was leaving I said, "Oh yes, don't forget the seedlings that I have in the car from the camp. There are three hemlock and one mountain laurel." She replied with a smile, "I'll keep them moist and in a cool place." She knew how I always liked to plant such seedlings from our travels, especially when we went to the mountains.

Dr. Ruffin Benton

Shortly thereafter, I was transferred. I was happy to get to the coronary care unit where Dr. Ruffin Benton came to see me. Dr. Benton is an easygoing, very polite man, obviously a well-trained family physician. He did a careful history and examination. He gathered important information about my past and about my family history. His examination was very thorough. He had a most pleasant bedside manner. He took all the time necessary to talk with me and my family. He answered all of Nez's questions and gave us plenty of time for discussion. He spent additional time talking with Betty, and although she does not encounter coronary heart disease in her pediatric practice, she was quite capable of understanding his findings and his plan of management.

I did not want to be my own physician or make all of the decisions about my management, but I did expect to be consulted, and Dr. Benton made this easy by requesting my input as to what we were to do next. We discussed alternatives. As soon as I had arrived and my electrocardiogram was found to be normal, I felt that an early catheterization would be required for a definitive diagnosis. He mentioned my being transported over to the heart unit in Asheville, North Carolina, where catheterization facilities were available. I felt quite comfortable, with no chest discomfort after the administration of the small single dose of Demerol. Together, we concluded that I would be observed overnight in the coronary care unit, and be reevaluated the following morning.

There were no serious problems during the night except for more of the abnormal beats such as those observed in the emergency room. Twice they set off the alarm, causing the intensive care nurses to rush to my bedside. Needless to say, this can create some degree of anxiety, particularly when the cardiologist-patient is observing his own monitor and appreciates the sometimes serious consequence of these observations.

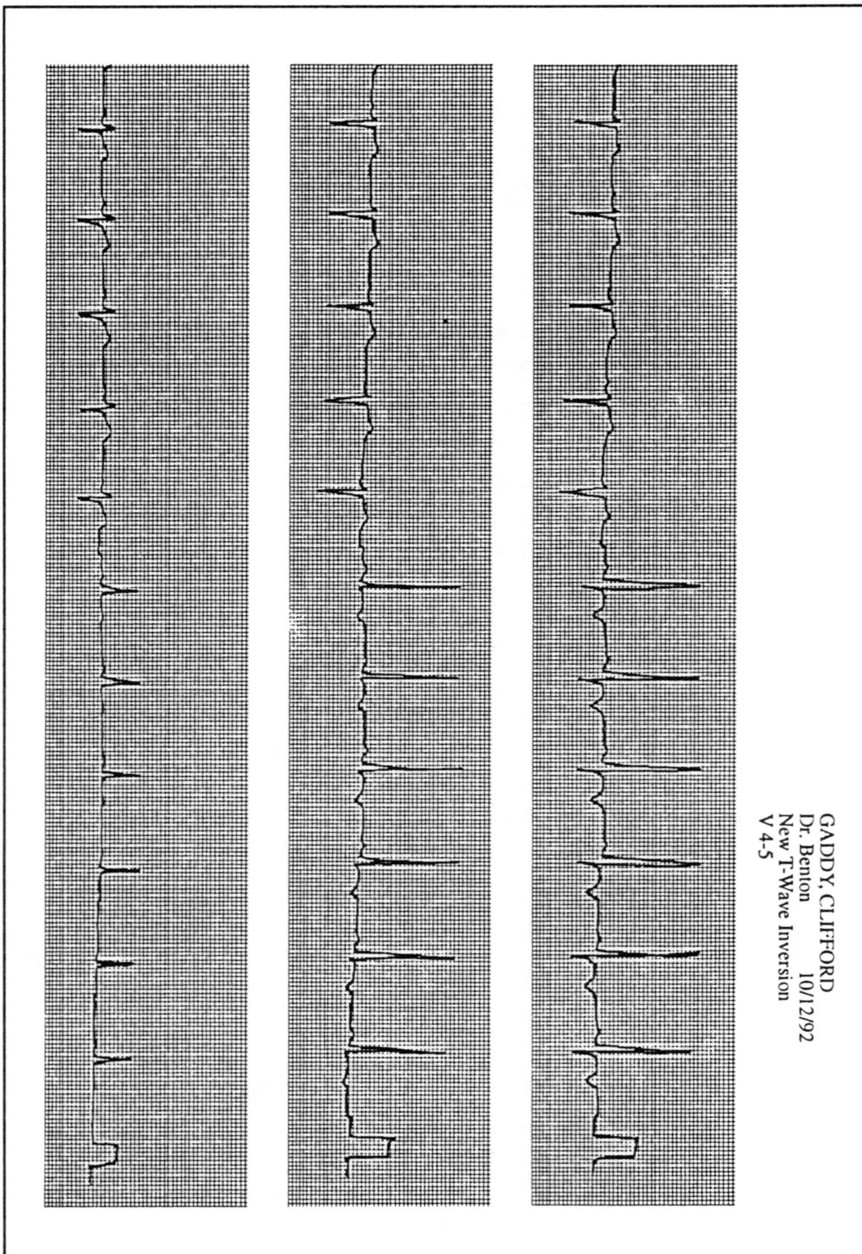

Figure 5. *Mild but significant changes in the author's EKG on the day after admission.*

We Choose Duke Medical Center

When Dr. Benton came in to see me on Monday morning, my electrocardiogram had been taken and definite abnormalities were now apparent. Fortunately, changes that would indicate a definite myocardial infarction (due to a coronary artery blood clot) were not present. They were mild, nonspecific changes, as noted on my tracing in figure 5. The T waves had become inverted (see the areas encircled by Dr. Benton). The tracing was taken from an area over the front of my heart. The changes were, in my mind, sufficient to conclude that my chest pains were associated with inadequate circulation and demanded further study.

Abnormal heartbeats continued to appear on the monitor, and, while there was no chest pain, it seemed obvious that further evaluation would be necessary. Dr. Benton suggested that I might have a cardiac ultrasound test done which was available on a portable ultrasound unit out of Asheville. We use this study commonly at home to help evaluate circulation to the heart muscle, but it seemed unlikely to me that this would provide a definitive answer in my particular circumstances. Further discussion of catheterization of the coronary arteries ensued.

Nez and I spent most of the day alone in the coronary care unit. I had a private room with a monitor. The nurses' station was across the hall. I could not have been treated more royally. All my needs were attended as promptly as possible. When I was served a meal there was always a guest tray for Nez. If I had a beverage she was offered one. In her absence the nurses told me how much they liked and admired her. This was probably because Nez, having been a nurse, was always very considerate. Never demanding, when I needed something she always made a pleasant request. Many patients and their families could take a lesson from her. An attitude of appreciation always seems to lead to better service.

Duke University Medical Center at Durham, North Carolina, was my logical choice for my catheterization. I have referred the largest share of my own patients needing heart surgery to Duke and to Bowman Gray Medical School in Winston-Salem, North Carolina.

Since Betty lives in Raleigh, North Carolina, and both Steve and Gary are in nearby Chapel Hill, Duke seemed the most practical choice. If I were to be kept at Duke for a period of time, this would give Nez a place to stay and the support she would need. Furthermore, Durham, North Carolina, is only an hour and fifteen minutes from our home in Danville, Virginia.

Life Flight

I asked Dr. Benton to discuss my transfer with Dr. Bob Califf of Duke Medical Center. The question arose as to how I should be transported. In the light of the potentially serious heart irregularities that I had observed on the monitor, I did not feel that Nez and I should make a five-hour drive to Durham unattended. We requested flight by helicopter. Dr. Benton and Dr. Califf discussed this and we were told that Life Flight, Duke's helicopter, would be leaving Durham in about an hour and would stop in Asheville for refueling. At this point we chose to have Nez go ahead and leave in her station wagon in order to arrive not long after our helicopter was to set down at Duke University Medical Center.

Before parting there in the coronary care unit at Brevard, I warned Nez that a helicopter flight from Brevard to Durham would be quite expensive, maybe as much as $4,000 or $5,000, to which she responded, "So what! Money is not worth anything unless you are here to spend it."

I hated to see Nez leave on her lonely trip. She insisted there would be no problem. She later told me that there had been a beautiful harvest moon to light her way, as if she had an angel riding alongside to guide her way.

The coronary care nurse advised me that a second intravenous infusion would be required prior to transport. She started another I.V. in my other arm. This was to guarantee ready access in the event of the development of a serious heart irregularity or cardiac arrest during transit. Should one I.V. become dislodged a backup would be available. Starting a new I.V. aboard the helicopter in flight would not be a simple task.

As I recall, at about 9:30 p.m., I could hear the loud engine as the helicopter approached the hospital landing pad. It was like hearing the siren of a life-saving ambulance or hearing Life Flight as it passed over our office building in Danville enroute for a medical center. Sometimes I would be aware of the specific patient being transported and how critically ill he was. The sound of the helicopter means that someone is in serious trouble.

By 10:00 p.m. I had been wheeled out on the stretcher and placed aboard the helicopter. I was riding up front in a semi-recumbent position just to the left of the pilot, where I could see everything. There was that bright full harvest moon. The sky was filled with stars. It would have been a great evening for anything except a trip to a medical center for a catheterization and possible heart surgery.

I was told that we reached a maximum cruising rate of 190 miles per hour. I had no chest discomfort throughout the flight. My blood pressure and my blood oxygen levels, which were being monitored periodically, were doing well. My heart beats were also being monitored. If there were any periods of irregularity, I was unaware of them, and none were reported to me.

Those of us who practice cardiology in Danville, Virginia, and commonly transfer patients for invasive procedures, have come to rely on the helicopter to get our patients promptly to the surrounding medical centers. The competent pilot and the coronary care nurses in attendance have made us feel confident about this mode of transportation in urgent situations.

I felt I was blessed to be flying during such a beautiful night with clear skies. Despite the noise of the engines and the uncertainty of the future, I was made to feel as secure as could be.

The Coronary Care Unit

We landed on the helicopter pad at Duke Medical Center at approximately midnight. I was pleased to see that Steve and Betty were waiting for me, along with a team of Duke's medical personnel. I was taken directly to the coronary care unit, where the portable monitoring units were switched with the monitors present at the bedside as well as at the nurses' station. It was gratifying to realize that I would no longer feel responsible for observing my own monitor.

Dr. Julie Fetters was my cardiologist. I had not previously met Dr. Fetters. I learned that she was a graduate of the Ohio State University College of Medicine and made her graduate cardiology studies at Duke Medical Center. We discussed how my pain had begun, and how I had been somewhat confused by the pains I had experienced in the past in my neck, shoulders, and arms. I told her of my treadmill stress test of eighteen months before, and how I had questioned its results. Of course, hindsight is better than foresight. She reviewed my chart records and examined my heart and lungs.

During the next hour, I must have been checked by half a dozen doctors, including cardiac fellows, residents, and students. Each followed an identical protocol. They might have referred to the three copies of my records that I brought from Brevard. Individually, each needed to know when my chest pain started, what it felt like, and how long it persisted, how much heart trouble my grandparents and parents had suffered, and about thirty other questions. They all listened to my heart, examined my lungs, and had me take a deep breath. All left without volunteering an opinion as to how they thought I was doing. I preferred to travel "incognito" and did not have M.D. by my name on my records or on my wrist bands. I thought I would like to see how the rest of the world was treated in this environment, and I must say I was favorably impressed at the way "Mr. Gaddy" was treated.

I am still somewhat uncertain as to whether being a physician relieved my anxiety, or whether knowing the potential hazards of what I was about to undergo increased it. I think that while I was a patient at Transylvania County Hospital, I felt somewhat more anxious because of my knowledge of potentially serious cardiac irregularities. In the Duke environment, I felt reassured by the knowledge that there were very competent people observing my monitor. I knew that personnel were available and prepared to take action should I develop ventricular fibrillation or cardiac arrest.

A study done several years ago evaluating the psychological effect on patients in the coronary unit who witnessed heart resuscitation on other patients in adjoining beds, reached a conclusion that surprised me. The majority of the patients reported a feeling of reassurance about resuscitation because of the seriousness of the efforts of the doctors, nurses, and the cardiopulmonary resuscitation team. I would have suspected that such an experience would leave a greater residue of anxiety than reassurance. One not so elderly patient said, "If they worked that hard to save the life of the little old man next to me, I know they would save me."

At about 3:00 a.m. an attractive young physician, who introduced herself as the intern, arrived. After about fifteen minutes of examination, her beeper went off and she asked to be excused to go to the emergency room, after which she came back and completed her examination. I was courteous and thanked her, because she may have been on duty for the past thirty-six hours with only brief naps in between. No doctor ever forgets his life as an intern!

The Catheterization Laboratory

Early on Tuesday morning, about six hours after my arrival at Duke, preparations were being made for my going to the catheterization lab to study my coronary arteries. The study was to be done by Dr. Robert (Jess) Peter. I had known Dr. Peter only by phone and correspondence. He is a very quiet and caring person who makes you feel comfortable in his presence. He asked if I had any questions. I was familiar with the procedure, but I welcomed the chance to have him review his plans with me. "It's the only way we can be sure of just what we are dealing with."

Certainly, in my case, there was no way of knowing whether I could be treated with a balloon dilatation catheter, coronary artery bypass grafts or even required to be on heart medications alone, without catheterization.

We were off to the catheterization laboratory. Nez, as always, was at my side. At the door to the lab she gave me a kiss and I could read the prayer on her lips. I had reassured her of the minimal hazard associated with the procedure, and Jess Peters had done likewise.

Cardiac catheterization is a much-utilized procedure today. A recent published survey showed that there were 1,402,700 catheterizations done on adults for angiograms in 1989. Without a doubt there were more in 1992. There are those who argue that there are too many studies done today, especially since thirty percent show perfectly normal angiograms. There is also the argument that so many catheterizations leads to an unnecessary number of bypass operations. Treadmill testing and other noninvasive procedures such as ultrasound or heart scanning techniques may obviate the need for catheterization in some instances. There was never any doubt in my mind about the absolute necessity for catheterization in my case.

What is known as a "sheath" was first introduced into my right femoral artery at the groin, after the area had been thoroughly sterilized with antiseptics. The insertion of the sheath, which is like a large needle, was done with a local anesthetic, so it caused no more discomfort than an injection of Novocain for a tooth to be extracted. Study of the heart and arteries was done by means of a liquid solution called contrast dye. Since body liquids, such as blood, do not create images on X-rays, a so-called contrast medium is injected to form a shadow of the interior of the heart and arteries. The catheter was introduced through the sheath up to my aorta, the large blood vessel originating from the heart. From here it was skillfully maneuvered into the tiny openings to the coronary blood vessels going to the heart muscle itself.

I am not sure if I was given any form of a tranquilizer. I was naturally concerned about what the findings might be, but I did not feel anxious about the procedure itself. I was wide awake and very alert. Dr. Peter described each part of the procedure as he performed it. From what my patients tell me, it is routine for everyone to be informed just as I was throughout the process.

A few ounces of contrast dye were injected into my heart to measure the exact amount of blood that was being pumped from my heart with each heartbeat. This is called "ejection fraction," a measurement of the percentage of the blood being pumped from the heart with each beat. Dr. Peter reported that my value was sixty-five percent, which is better than that of the average person my age. This, of course, was very reassuring. Those with low percentage outputs have weak hearts, and generally do poorly even after successful surgery.

I was warned about the intense flushing that occurs along with each injection of the dye, and now I know what it is like for a woman to have severe "hot flashes."

Risk during catheterization in the hands of an expert like Dr. Peter is minimal. Dislodgment of a cholesterol fragment from the aorta by the catheter may cause a stroke or heart attack, but such is a very rare occurrence. Mortality in experienced laboratories is reported to be less than one in 2,500 tests. Bleeding around the site of the introduction of the catheter in the groin sometimes occurs, but is rarely of serious consequence. Discoloration around the puncture site due to a small amount of bleeding under the skin is not uncommon.

The Coronary Angiograms

The angiograms are the pictures of the coronary arteries made when the dye is injected into them and an X-ray is done. A small catheter was introduced into each of my major coronary arteries. First, a picture of the right coronary artery was reproduced. It showed a ninety-five percent restriction at one point and seventy-five percent at another. Next were the two major branches of the left coronary artery. These were the anterior descending branch, which was also restricted by ninety-five percent at two points, and the circumflex branch, which was narrowed by seventy-five percent at two areas. The ramus is a small and short branch off the anterior descending artery. It was narrowed by ninety-five percent. A schematic drawing of my coronary arteries as they appear in the angiography report is seen in figure 6.

The X-ray monitor was moved within my view. Jess showed me the defects right there in the cath lab, and immediately concluded that I would do best if I had three bypass grafts done. I was told that the ramus would not be grafted because of its small size. I was pleased that I didn't have to endure a long period of suspense to learn the results of the study and what my treatment was to be. Naturally, I was disappointed that my angiograms showed more extensive blockage so that I could not have balloon dilatation of the defects done. This would have enabled me to go home in twenty-four hours and back to work in a week. Balloon dilatation (PTCA—see below) is most successful if the narrowed segment is very short. Nevertheless, I returned to my room feeling good, believing that with three successful grafts, my heart would be significantly better than it had been for the past year or longer.

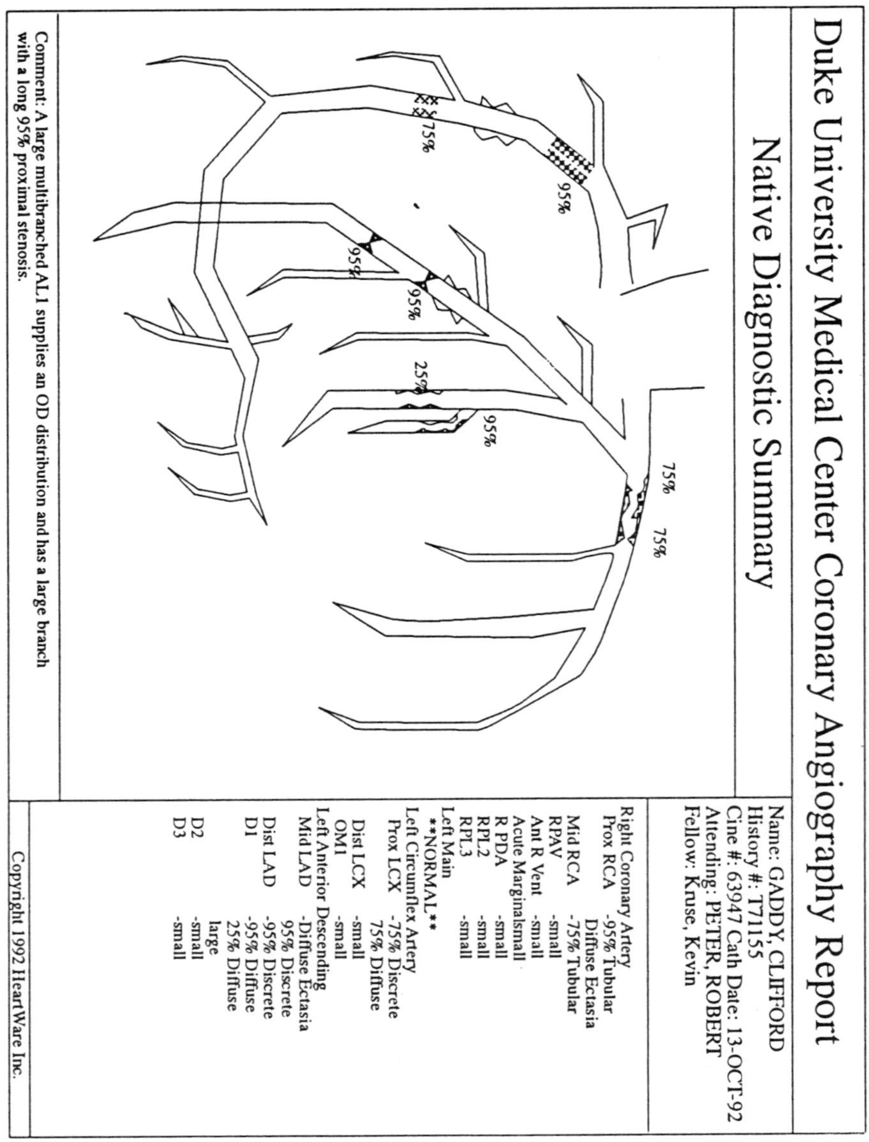

Duke University Medical Center Coronary Angiography Report

Native Diagnostic Summary

Name: GADDY, CLIFFORD
History #: T71155
Cine #: 63947 Cath Date: 13-OCT-92
Attending: PETER, ROBERT
Fellow: Kruse, Kevin

Right Coronary Artery
Prox RCA -95% Tubular
Diffuse Ectasia
Mid RCA -75% Tubular
RPAV -small
Ant R Vent -small
Acute Marginalsmall
R PDA -small
RPL2 -small
RPL3 -small
Left Main
NORMAL
Left Circumflex Artery
Prox LCX -75% Discrete
75% Diffuse
Dist LCX -small
OM1 -small
Left Anterior Descending
Mid LAD -Diffuse Ectasia
95% Discrete
Dist LAD -95% Discrete
D1 -95% Diffuse
25% Diffuse
large
D2 -small
D3 -small

Comment: A large multibranched AL1 supplies an OD distribution and has a large branch with a long 95% proximal stenosis.

Figure 6. *Author's angiographic report showing six areas of major obstruction (seventy-five percent or greater).*

I still wondered about the small ramus artery, narrowed by ninety-five percent. Was it possible that Jess would leave that little artery unrepaired to ensure that I would not get back on the high-wire rope course again?

Collateral Circulation

When there is a partial blockage in one of the coronary arteries, there appears to be an effort on the part of the body to improve its own circulation past this point of narrowing. We call this "collateral circulation." With two of my three major coronary arteries blocked ninety-five percent and the third being blocked seventy-five percent, it would appear impossible for me to have carried on anything like normal physical activity if I had not had significant collateral vessels to develop. I am confident now that for many months I had been having anginal pains. When walking up rather steep grades carrying my golf bag, carrying one end of a railroad tie (for flower-bed borders and such), and digging or moving rocks, I observed chest pains that I now firmly recognize as originating with my heart. I presume that such strenuous activity on a regular basis had enabled me to build collateral arteries that had bypassed the points of obstruction.

Were it not for collateral circulation, I think I never could have reached the level of the high wire, let alone complete the rope walk. If the total circulation to my heart muscle depended on what was being carried only through the three major arteries, I am sure I could not have done it.

There is evidence that those individuals who have narrowing of circulation in the legs are able to improve their exercise capacity through a program of enforced walking. On such a program, one walks as much as possible, constrained only by the degree of pain in his legs. With continued effort we know that ultimately many such individuals are able to walk a longer time and greater distances before being limited by the pain (called claudication). These findings have a significant bearing on the importance of a program of cardiac rehabilitation following coronary bypass surgery or balloon dilatation of the coronary arteries. The same can be said about those patients who have suffered a heart attack with a blood clot, who may not have had an invasive procedure such as bypass surgery or balloon dilatation. Of course, as I will emphasize later, such a program must be tailored for the given individual and carried out under careful supervision.

Percutaneous Transluminal Coronary Angioplasty

Percutaneous transluminal coronary angioplasty sounds exceptionally complex, but is merely a descriptive term. Usually we abbreviate it: PTCA. It is the procedure in which a cardiac surgeon takes a small catheter with a balloon tip and introduces it through the skin, into the femoral artery up to the aorta and into the coronary arteries, much as is done during the catheterization study to insert dye for the angiograms. In PTCA, however, the balloon catheter is introduced into the narrowed coronary artery and is then inflated, making it possible to compress the cholesterol plaques that are causing the obstruction. Upon removal of the balloon, the blood vessel is left with a larger diameter. This procedure is done without having to enter the chest cavity surgically and therefore is a significantly easier and less traumatic procedure for the patient. It is done while the patient remains awake. If it can be done successfully, the patient can usually be out of the hospital in a couple of days, and often is able to resume work in a week or ten days.

Only certain patients are candidates for balloon angioplasty because of the nature of the narrowing in the coronary arteries. Unless the narrowing is rather localized, the balloon therapy may not be suitable. This is why I was not a suitable candidate. One must also remember that there will occasionally be a tear in the coronary artery when the balloon is dilated, likely requiring immediate coronary artery bypass surgery. For this reason the procedure is advocated only in an institution where bypass surgery is available. Also of significant concern is the fact that approximately one-third of the patients who have balloon dilatation will require a repeat treatment in three to six months. Sometimes several dilatations are required.

The fact that repeat dilatations are routinely necessary has discouraged some patients. I have attended patients who have required two and three repeat dilatations. With persistence, however, a long-lasting result can often be achieved.

On Tuesday afternoon I called back to my office to report on my catheterization. When I talked with Dr. Edwin Harvie, my partner in practice since 1964, I learned that Dr. Peter had already called to discuss the angiographic findings with him. Dr. Harvie quoted Dr. Peter as being "ecstatic" about the findings, feeling that my report was compatible with excellent results from bypass surgery.

I had been taking a blood thinner called Heparin. For this reason I had to maintain complete immobility of my right leg for four hours after the catheter was removed, and an additional four hours after the sheath was removed. Without a doubt, this was the most difficult part of the catheterization procedure. Most of the time Nez was there to keep her hand on my foot to be sure I did not forget. Betty and Janet were there some of the time to warn me.

Seven and three-quarter hours after the procedure, I needed to get to the bathroom to eliminate some of the copious intravenous fluid I had been receiving. The nurse caught me in the act, and I was chastised for getting up ahead of schedule. I apologized, for I really didn't want to be guilty of breaking rules. I dislike having patients break rules. Nurses at the Memorial Hospital in Danville often chuckle at me when they call to report that a patient has violated some rule, such as getting out of bed too early. When it will not endanger the patient, I reply, "I can't tolerate patients who don't follow rules, so change the rules. Write an order for him to be up as desired!"

Emotional Responses to the Attack

I experienced a variety of emotional responses, especially during the first few days after my attack.

Denial was first. I tried to ignore the chest pain I experienced while I was playing tennis on the first day at camp and while I vigorously paddled the white-water rapids in the canoe on the second day. Certainly, the pain I experienced on the high-wire rope walk was coming from my heart. Because the pain was atypical, I pretended it was not my heart although I knew it had to be. Denial is not an unusual reaction in many patients with chest pain. It is common for patients to fail to get early thrombolytic (clot-dissolving) treatment, which can preserve heart function and save one's life—all due to denial.

Anxiety and *fear* cannot be denied while I was in pain on the high-wire rope. Unfortunately, these emotions were not strong enough to overcome my desire to complete the course. It surely would have been to my advantage to have swallowed my pride, acknowledged my well-founded fear, and asked to be brought down from the high wire at any point during the walk.

I have felt some degree of *humiliation* and *resentment,* especially in dealing with patients and some friends who ask, "Why have you not been practicing what you have been advising us?" Without knowing that there are factors beyond our usual control, such as genetic problems, they assumed I was less faithful to the usual risk factors than I ought to have been.

Needless to say, in the light of these other strong emotional responses, there was some *depression* as well. Depression, it is now clear, is more than a mere reaction to other emotional factors. Duke

Medical Center and other institutions are currently evaluating this problem that seems to be more pronounced in older patients and seems to correlate with the duration on the cardiopulmonary bypass machine.

There seems to also be a relationship between the degree of depression and social support for the patient. This may be why depression was less of a problem for me than for many others: through it all, I had the constant and strong support and encouragement of Nez and our whole family.

During the early days I felt a certain amount of *anger*. I felt I did not deserve my condition. I had many patients and a number of friends my age whose health habits were far worse than mine. So I asked, "Why me?"

"Why Me?"

This thought entered my mind a great deal soon after the attack of pain and the confirmation of serious coronary disease. I had worked to avoid coronary heart disease. For many years we have avoided cholesterol and saturated fats in our diet. My midday snack at the office has often been an apple, or popcorn without salt or butter. At home, Nez, having been a nurse and a dietitian, rarely serves eggs, cheese, pork, or dark meats, and I nearly always avoid them when eating away from home.

Tobacco has never been a part of my life. As I grew up, my father strongly condemned tobacco, although he himself smoked. He promised me that if I did not start smoking before the age of twenty-one he would give me a gold watch. I was only fifteen when he died, but my mother gave me his watch, which I treasure to this day. I never have bought a package of cigarettes for my own use.

Thirty to forty years ago it was a tradition to hand out cigars on having a new baby. This happened often at our house (six children) and I smoked a few of the leftovers with my friends, but I never bought a box for my own use. I was happy to see the tradition of cigars to celebrate new babies fall by the wayside.

Exercise has been easy for me because I have always been an outdoorsman. Growing and transplanting trees, moving stones, and using a chainsaw have been fun for me. Walking and carrying my golf clubs has been the rule for me through the years. The immediate effect of some forms of exercise has been to cause hurting in my neck, but the long-term effect may have been helpful. I have felt that the exercise in which I have engaged has strengthened my heart and improved my collateral coronary circulation. I cannot honestly say when, or how much of, my neck, shoulder, and chest pain began manifesting angina.

High blood pressure occurs in my family. I have effectively controlled my blood pressure with low-dose medication and dietary salt restriction.

I have learned through scientific testing that I qualify as a "hyperreactor" to acute stress, with increased heart rate and elevated blood pressure, especially the latter. This was established by cardiovascular monitoring during a timed examination of problem solving. This study was performed on volunteers at the meeting of the American College of Cardiology in 1986. The role of chronic stress in sustained hypertension is suspected, but less well established.

Stress is always included as an important factor in the development of coronary artery heart disease. Its effect is less well documented than that of cholesterol and tobacco use. We often have little control over certain stress factors, but control over our diets and the use of tobacco products is our own responsibility.

Any individual who withstands the rigorous training required to become a doctor knows about stress. I started school at age five and graduated from high school at sixteen. Because of World War II, training was accelerated, and I did not have a summer recess throughout ten years of premedical, medical, and graduate studies. The competition to qualify for admission to medical school was intense. After admission it became greater. I will never forget the orientation lecture by the late dean of admissions at Bowman Gray School of Medicine, Dr. Hubert Vann: "Gentlemen, look in front and on either side of yourself. Next year one of you will not be here." Dr. Vann pointed out that the school had accepted twenty percent more students than it could accommodate during the last three years of medical school. I have always felt that such a policy was cruel and unnecessary punishment. Today, I understand this policy has changed and everyone who is admitted is expected to become a physician.

The practice of medicine has had its long hours and stressful times for me. This was especially true in the days of my solo practice, my first twelve years of work in Danville. Yet I found it so satisfying that it did not seem stressful. One of our children often rode along when I made home calls. Patients still remind me of this today. For example, I sometimes hear, "I understand the little girl who came with you to my house twenty-five years ago is now a pediatrician." Appreciation for my services was great. Sometimes the compensation was a bushel of apples just picked from the orchard, or a fresh tenderloin steak. In those days almost no one had medical insurance but no inquiry about compensation was made. For rural patients payment was often made when the seasons' crops were sold. I had no liability insurance and no thought of any form of litigation ever passed through my mind. It was a great era in which to practice medicine. Many forms of stress that we have today did not exist.

After the development of pains in my neck and arms from the old injury, life in general, became more stressful. Recreation was limited. I gave up tennis. Jogging aggravated the discomfort. I did not give up golf but for a while I played wearing a soft collar around my neck. It worsened my golf handicap, but then it never was very good anyway. The most distressing part of my malady was the interference with my work. Being unable to rest at night made coping with long hours in the emergency room and coronary care unit near impossible. This led me to request a less strenuous course that exempted me from hospital work and night call. I requested to become a member of the hospital's Courtesy Staff. I was never as happy with the limited role but I had no other reasonable option. I was sometimes made to feel less important to the practice. This was not a satisfying feeling although patients were very understanding.

My point is that *stress* is directly related to your *attitude* toward the challenges you face.

A greater risk factor, I believe, resides in the *genes*. We will discuss this in greater detail later on.

Support Groups

I have been asked by a number of people about the level of fear that I had with the onset of my chest pain and the subsequent catheterization and surgery. Generally speaking, I was somewhat astounded at the degree of calm I experienced throughout the entire procedure. I believe the greatest feeling of security comes from the people who care the most for you. The greatest comfort came from having Nez always available for me. She is not an emotional person, and her stability offered me a lot of reassurance. She was always there and accompanied me to the door of the cath lab and to the door of the operating room, and was there to see me out each time. There was so much support from my entire family that I feel confident this helped allay fears that I otherwise might have have had.

I also think there is a feeling of satisfaction in the achievements of your family, of whom you are very proud, so that even under hazardous circumstances, you have an underlying sense of accomplishment. What I am trying to say, is that I feel my life has been very satisfying. Of course, there are still lots of things out there that I want to achieve and a lot of pleasures that I anticipate. But life has been so fulfilling that I haven't had time for the dread of dying.

Family support is more than just being there. It is a feeling that has developed through time. I have seen many families cluster around a patient in time of crisis when I was confident that some of it was out of a feeling of guilt. We physicians recognize them. They appear often at the time of a terminal event and make unreasonable demands, often overruling family members who have cared for the patient for months or years. It often appears that they are reacting to their own feelings of neglect of the patient in the past. This is not the kind of support I had from my family. I have often thought and sometimes expressed, "They are not only my family; they are my very best friends."

I would not want to deceive you into believing there was no anxiety while I was in the emergency room at Transylvania County Hospital and was observing a monitor that showed frequent abnormal heartbeats and brief runs of a rhythm that may be a forerunner of what we call ventricular tachycardia. I had to try to conceal my anxiety. Once my pain was relieved and my heart rhythm became regular, and I had someone in whom I had great confidence to observe my monitor, I felt much more at ease.

I had an early call from Dr. Robert Setzer, pastor of the First Baptist Church in Danville, asking if he might come to see me. I realized he had just recently arrived in Danville and that there was much he needed to do. I said to him, "Bob, you have a lot to do at the church and it would be a three-hour round-trip for you to come to Durham. I will accept this call by telephone as a visit from you if you have other things that you feel you ought to be doing."

Nevertheless, I was quite happy to see Bob and his wife Bambi, a portrait artist, arrive at the foot of my bed. His prayer was most welcome and comforting. I must say I had a rather eerie feeling because it had been just a short time before when I attended a funeral service I thought Bob had conducted beautifully, and in jest I commented, "Bob, I liked your service and I want you to stick around to do my funeral service."

Of course, I thought I was in excellent health and the comment was only intended as a compliment. I could not help but wonder if he was also thinking about this as he stood before me, knowing that I faced heart surgery with its hazards the next day.

I also had a call from our former pastor, Dr. Luke Smith, who is now in Richmond, Virginia. He and Janie came to see me shortly after my return to Danville, bringing a copy of C. S. Lewis's book *Surprised by Joy.* Another former pastor, Dr. Robert Forehand, also called, as did so many other friends offering prayers and support. I am confident this was important in my feeling of assurance of my recovery.

The Sunday school group to which I am very devoted offered a great deal of support with phone calls, cards, and visits. Their assurances of concern and their prayers were gratifying.

Members of the Rotary Club of Danville is a group with whom I feel a close relationship. I heard from many of them and their support meant a good deal.

My regular golf-foursome partners, Bob Adams, George Shields, and Clif Plowden, showed up at my bedside on the afternoon before surgery. I had to appreciate their concern because it was such a beautiful day outside for golf.

Vic Cresenzo and his son Mark, both physicians, came to see me. Vic has had considerable experience as a clinical cardiologist for forty years. Further, over the past fourteen years, he has had coronary bypass surgery on two occasions, a valve replacement, and a permanent pacemaker implanted. Our associations in medical school, postgraduate training, and recertification examinations have made us and our families very close. He and Fran have five sons. Vic has great determination and capacity to bounce back. I hope to maintain his kind of determination. He, also, has a very supporting family.

Nez's friends Mary Lou Barr and Helen Petty came to provide support for her during my stay in the operating room and cardiac recovery. The knowledge that Nez had the support she needed was helpful to me.

My partner in practice Dr. Edwin Harvie also paid me a visit. We had previously talked on the phone. We have had an outstanding relationship for the nearly twenty-nine years we have been associated. He brought me good wishes from all of our office personnel and from a number of friends and patients. Naturally, this made me feel better. He had discussed my angiograpic findings with Dr. Peter and brought me encouragement about the prospects of excellent surgical results.

Dr. Robert Jones talked to me about my surgery and explained that because I was in good physical condition, my mortality rate from surgery should be less than one to two percent. Although I was already aware of the statistical facts, it was helpful to talk to him and appreciate how the data applied directly to me. Lurking in the back of my mind was the question, “Could I be one of those in the one to two percent?” I remember a professor of surgery in medical school who used to say, “If your patient is in that tiny minority group it becomes one hundred percent for him.” In the past I have been the one presenting the information about prognosis rather than being the recipient. The facts were very reassuring.

I jokingly commented that the greatest risk probably was getting on the Durham freeway to Interstate 40 and up State Route 86 and arriving safely back in Danville.

To the Operating Room

The Scrub Down

When I was aroused on Thursday morning, the first order of business was the "scrub down". The nurse came in with the container of liquid antiseptic soap, and set about to scrub me down and shave me from my Adam's apple to my toes. I was covered with sterile drapes and put on a stretcher. I was ready to head out to the operating suite.

On to the Operating Room

Support was always near. Nez never left my side. She was there to massage my neck and back as she has so frequently done since my neck injury years ago. More important, she was there to reassure me. All of the adult members of the family who were with us at Camp Eagle's Nest were on hand the day of my surgery.

Our oldest son Cliff was not present because of his work with Brookings Institute in Washington, D.C. He earned his doctorate from Duke University a year and a half ago. His degree was in Russian Economics and he had just returned from Russia a few days earlier. This had been his fourth trip to Russia in recent months. His wife Kerstin, a Swedish girl, earned her master's in German from Duke at the same time, and is now seeking her Ph.D. from Georgetown University, where she is teaching German to undergraduates. Cliff, having objected to participation in the Vietnam War, had spent seventeen years in Stockholm, and he and Kerstin have been back in this country for five years. They have two children, ages six and four.

We requested that Bobby and Evelyn not come from Gloucester because we appreciated the fact that they were quite busy. Bobby is a skilled craftsman who makes fine furniture. Together they are woodcutters for a nationally renowned artist in Yorktown, Virginia. Their Christmas ornaments have been selected by the Museum of American Folk Art in New York and have adorned the official White House tree during the Reagan years. They were quite involved in preparation of colonial toys and decorative carvings for the oncoming Christmas season. Evelyn vowed to come on my return home to be of help.

I was scheduled for early surgery so I was near the front of the line. Nez described the line of stretchers waiting for entry into the operating room as being like the planes lined up on a runway at Chicago-O'Hare International Airport! She made it easier for me by her calm demeanor and lack of emotion. She added confidence to my guarded feeling that everything was sure to go all right. I knew she was following the admonition of the Apostle Paul when he said, "Pray without ceasing." This was what I was doing until the anesthetic took effect.

When I entered the operating room, I was surrounded by unknowns. They were all so well draped and masked that they had to reintroduce themselves to me one by one. I had no problem recognizing Dr. Jones by his voice. His assistant was Dr. Kevin P. Landolfo, and my anesthesiologist was Dr. Fiona M. Clements. There must have been a half dozen nurses on hand, but I couldn't begin to remember their names. Any of the whole group could have easily managed a bank holdup without ever being recognized!

Thoughts That Pass through Your Mind

At a time like this, when you are entering the operating room, a lot of thoughts pass through your mind in a short time.

I thought about my living will, a document I so often talk about to patients and their families. Often it is for people in a nursing home or those preparing to go. I knew my living will was prepared and signed, but gave little thought that it could ever be needed by me. In any event, I knew that Nez was aware of how each of us felt about the use of life-sustaining measures beyond hope. I saw no reason to discuss the will at this particular time.

I thought about my parents and their ambitions for me. I can't remember when I didn't want to become a doctor. I must have been in elementary school when I ordered from a magazine a copy of a book called *The Modern Home Physician*. I had answers to medical problems that other kids didn't know. I honestly cannot say whether the idea to become a doctor originated with me or whether it was a reflection of my parents' desire. My father had said that if it was necessary to sell the family farm in order for me to go to medical school he would do so. Fortunately, the necessity never arose.

When I was growing up on the farm in South Carolina, it was my job to help slop the pigs, as well as to feed the chickens and throw hay to the cows. If there was a "runt" pig in the litter rejected by the sow, it was my job to adopt the little fellow and feed him until he was able to fend for himself. Likewise, if a chicken was hit by an automobile on the road, it was I who would splint the leg and look after it until it healed. I wanted to look after the ailing animals, and perhaps this had something to do with my father's ambition that I become a physician. Unfortunately, he died when I was fifteen years old and he was never to know that his wish came true. As for the farm animals, I can still remember how I used to run and hide when my dad was ready to slaughter a young steer for beef, or slaughter the hogs for pork, which we consumed throughout the winter. I even hated to see my mother wring the neck of a chicken on Saturday afternoon, but it did not keep me from reaching for the drumstick when it had been fried on Sunday.

I thought about some of the specific patients I have attended over the years. You can't help but remember some of those who expressed a feeling of dependence upon you. You have treated them so many times over a period of two or three decades. I guess every doctor who has practiced for a long time has been asked not to retire while a long-standing patient is still around. It gives you a strange feeling to realize that an unforeseen event might abruptly interrupt such a relationship.

The Bypass Operation

The Miraculous Heart-Lung Machine

Any time during surgery on the heart, whether it is interior, such as replacing or repairing a heart valve, or exterior, as in a coronary-artery bypass operation, a cardiopulmonary bypass machine (commonly called the heart-lung machine) must be connected to the patient to take over the function of the heart and lungs. Blood returning to the right side of the heart, which is low in oxygen, is diverted to the machine, where it passes through an oxygenator that adds oxygen to the red blood cells and at the same time removes carbon dioxide. Then by means of a pump that takes over the normal action of the heart, it is forced through a filter and into a heat exchanger. This unit cools the blood so as to lower the body temperature, slowing metabolism and thus allowing more time for performing the operation. This same unit will warm the blood when the operation is complete. The blood now returns to the aorta, which is the large blood vessel coming from the heart, which delivers it to the brain and to the remainder of the body's vital organs. A clamp is placed between the heart and the beginning of the aorta so that the heart can now be isolated from the circulation and surgery on the coronary arteries can begin. A cardioplegic (literally "heart-paralyzing") solution stops the heart's effort to beat, and the grafts are put in place.

A segment of vein is taken from the leg and is sewn between the aorta and the defective artery just beyond the point of obstruction. A bypass is put in place at each obstructed coronary artery. In my case, as was indicated by the angiogram report, there were three grafts inserted. Two used veins from the leg and the third used the internal mammary artery. At this point the cardioplegic solution is removed, rewarming is begun, and the aorta is unclamped. To initiate the normal heart beat, an electrical shock is sometimes applied to the heart muscle. Occasionally, a pacemaker is implanted to maintain a regular heart beat. This is generally a temporary pacemaker which can be removed before hospital discharge. In my case, my heart resumed its own beat without such assistance.

The whole idea of the heart-lung machine boggles my mind. It is almost like trying to understand how a computer works. It is much too complex for me. It has been developed over a period of years to a point of near perfection. It astounds me to appreciate the fact that my heart was totally inactive, not beating at all, while it was being repaired, and yet the rest of my body, including my brain and other vital organs, were being sustained by a machine. Management of the bypass machine is a science in itself. A great deal of training is required. Supervision of the machine is a very critical part of the coronary bypass procedure.

A friend of mine who has had heart surgery on three different occasions shares in my amazement. He says, in jest, "Any skilled Chinese seamstress could do the operation, but the heart-lung machine is the working of many geniuses."

The Wounds

Apart from the sites of many needles and tubes there are only two wounds in a coronary bypass operation.

The Sternum. Opening the breast bone (sternum) is done from the top to the bottom so that the ribs can be spread wide to give ready access to the heart for the surgeon. For this they use a sophisticated oscillating saw (known as the Stryker saw), carefully maneuvered to divide the sternum without injuring any organs within the chest.

The Veins. The veins are removed from the leg by one single long incision, in a procedure similar to what was used thirty or forty years ago for removal of varicose veins. The surgeon who removes the vein has an important task. It was learned many years ago, when bypass surgery was in its infancy, that meticulous handling of the vein was important to help protect against any injury that might cause it to block. Unfortunately, some patients with varicosities had the veins stripped out in order to overcome the stagnation of venous blood in these vessels, only to learn in later years that the veins were no longer available as grafts for bypass surgery. I have had at least one such patient in my practice.

When veins are put in place to bypass the coronary artery obstruction, they are placed in reverse. That is, they are placed "upside down" so that the valves which were important in allowing blood to flow upward in the legs back to the heart will not block forward flow in the coronary arteries.

Many patients of mine report that they feel more discomfort from the incision in the leg where the vein is removed than from that in the sternum. Not so in my case. When I was growing up on the farm, I used to get as bad a pain produced by a laceration from climbing through a barbed wire fence (especially if the bull was after me), than I did from my vein surgery. Occasionally inadvertent injury to a saphenous nerve, which lies adjacent to the saphenous vein (chief superficial leg vein), will lead to prolonged discomfort in this area.

It is important to protect the incision from trauma and I have found that the use of an elastic (Ace) bandage or compression hose can afford protection and help avoid swelling.

The sternal wound was more uncomfortable. For two weeks, it was quite painful to cough, sneeze, or even laugh. Some of my patients and friends who have had the procedure suggest that the wires used to hold the sternum back together were not tight enough.

(I have thought about devising a pair of pliers that has a torque-wrench effect so that we can get just the right amount of tension on those wires when the patient is put back together. I would like someone who knows mechanics and is familiar with patents to get in touch with me.)

The skin over the sternum may remain sensitive to touch for some time, and I found a soft cotton-lined apparel, such as an athletic sweatshirt, most comfortable. Some patients continue to complain of pain over the sternum. I have one patient who after two years continues to ask for a permit from me for the Division of Motor Vehicles exempting him from the use of his automobile seat belt.

I have had one patient who has had nonunion of his sternal incision. He is now a nursing home patient who is not competent to tell me why this happened. It most likely came as a consequence of lifting prior to adequate healing of the breastbone. It apparently is no longer uncomfortable. It acts as a hinge as he breaths and undoubtedly creates a small amount of inefficiency in his respirations. Knowledge of this complication made me more cognizant of the need to avoid lifting early after surgery.

Patients have to be careful about development of infection in the skin along the incision sites, both in the leg and sternum, but I experienced no problem of this sort.

I have had a few individuals who suffered irritation of the sternal incision, due to failure of the interior stitches to absorb in a normal fashion. These have required removal as they worked their way to the skin. Except for inconvenience, this problem is of no consequence.

I was put back together at the skin level with a sophisticated staple gun. I couldn't resist counting the staples. From the two incisions combined, I had 58 staples. The cardiac resident, Dr. Ronald Lilly, who removed them, presented them to me. I thought maybe I could devise a necklace for one of my granddaughters, but so far I have not been able to figure out how to do this. If someone has a suggestion, I would like to hear it. They ought to be recycled, since they were probably more expensive than most semi-precious stones.

The Bypass Grafts

The number of grafts done at the time of surgery obviously will vary depending on the results of the angiograms. Sometimes as many as five or more grafts may be done. I had three, which is about the usual number. (See figure 7.)

Veins taken from the legs were used for two of the grafts: the right coronary artery (A) and the circumflex artery (B).

The third graft was done with the internal mammary artery (C). This artery lies behind the breastbone and is readily accessible for

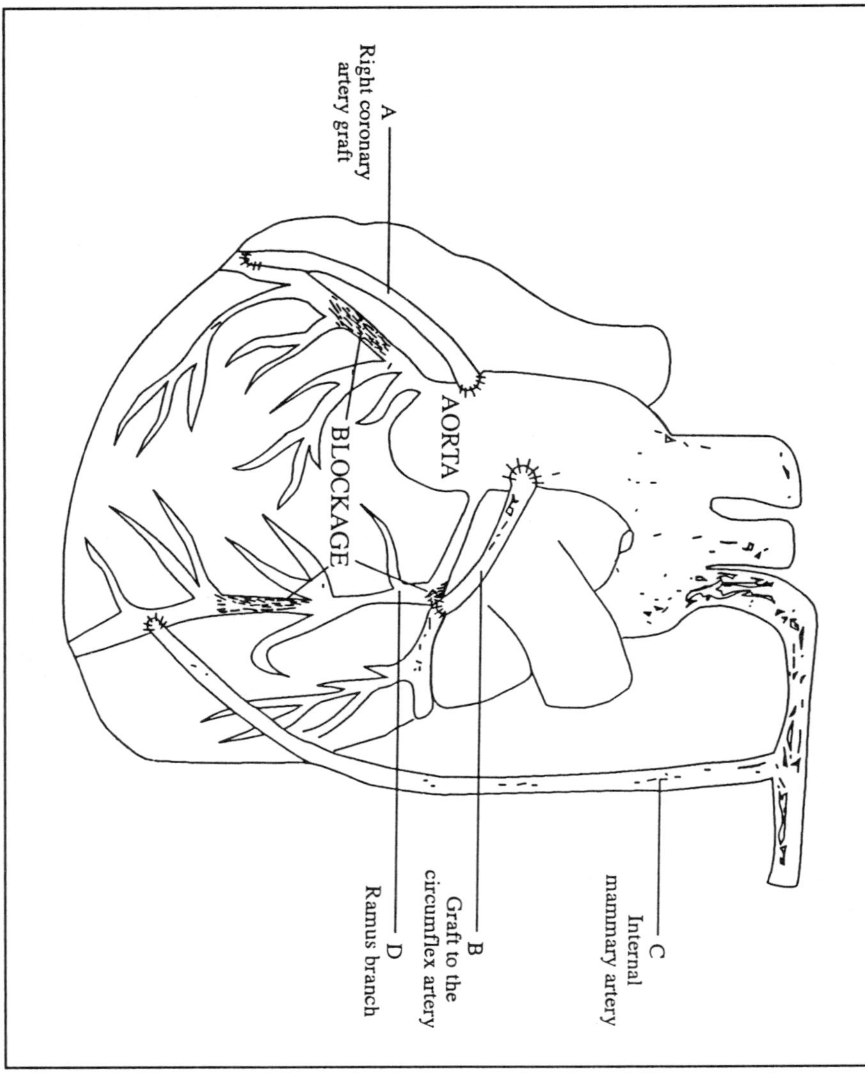

Figure 7. *Diagram of the author's three grafts. A and B show saphenous vein grafts; C is a graft from the internal mammary artery.*

attachment to one of the major coronary arteries. In my case, it was attached to the anterior descending artery.

With the use of the internal mammary artery, the greatest success is achieved in establishing a conduit that is least likely to undergo closure. Closures are nearly five times greater with vein grafts than with arterial grafts. The internal mammary artery is the choice vessel for grafting in all cases, but is especially useful in individuals seventy years and older. Anginal pain has returned in less than half the number of patients following an arterial graft as compared to a vein graft. Death due to heart causes is proportionally reduced in those whose internal mammary arteries were used for bypass grafts.

The Ramus branch (D), which is small and short, was ninety-five percent occluded in my case, but was not grafted. It was felt unnecessary to do so because of its small size.

The Cardiac Recovery Room

The night following my surgery was spent in the surgical intensive care unit. I must have slept a good deal, for I don't remember experiencing much pain. The greatest frustration came when I was recovering from the anesthetic. I had a tube through my mouth into my wind pipe. This is called an endotrachial tube. I could not talk, so I could not ask questions.

As I was being weaned off the respirator, it was important for me to voluntarily breathe deeply in order to keep my blood oxygen level in a suitable range. This is how it is determined that the respirator is no longer needed and the tube is ready to be removed. I remember the nurse who cared for me throughout the night saying, "Dr. Gaddy, stay awake and breathe hard. Your oxygen level is too low." I cooperated the best I could, but would soon drop back off to sleep and he would awaken me again. I had one free hand and I found that I could keep myself awake better if I slapped my thigh repeatedly and painfully to keep from going back to sleep. I think this must have been an original technique because it created a bit of interest when I would periodically slap myself, making a noise heard across the unit. It was a welcome relief to have the tube removed.

We who practice the medical arts are often accused of using vague terms that can't be understood. This may be generally true, but I can point out one exception. As I was coming out of the twilight zone I found myself standing by the bedside with the nurse holding the urinal. She didn't ask me if I would urinate or if I would void. All I can remember her saying was, "Pee, Dr. Gaddy, pee." How could she be more explicit than that? Confused or not, I knew what she wanted me to do and I did it.

Throughout the night blood samples were taken from my "central venous catheter," located in the small chamber of the right side of my heart. Measurements of my blood oxygen level, the blood pH, potassium, and other chemistries, which can be altered by the heart-lung machine or surgery, were done. Critical pressure readings were also taken to evaluate heart function and the need for more or less intravenous fluids.

I later learned that I had some periods of confusion during the night. I am sure it was a busy evening for my attendants but I can recall very little.

Tubes and More Tubes

When you return from the operating room, you may be surprised at the number of tubes inserted in your body. I had infusion tubes going into both of my arms. There was also the central venous catheter into my right jugular vein and hence to my vena cava. The purpose of this one was to constantly monitor pressures, electrolytes, blood chemistries, oxygen, blood pH, and blood cell levels. In fact, I think almost anything you wanted to know about my body you could have determined by getting a blood sample from this tube.

One tube was left in the artery to my lungs to monitor pressure there for a while after surgery was complete. When I awoke there was a garden-hose-size tube that passed through my mouth that I knew went into my trachea (windpipe), to which the respirator was attached. There was an indwelling catheter in my urinary bladder to measure my fluid output via the kidneys.

When my chest dressings subsequently were removed, I found three tubes coming out of my chest wall. One was in my left lung cavity, one in the right lung cavity, and the third in my heart cavity. This was in the pericardial sack that surrounds the heart and required opening to approach the arteries that were bypassed. These were all to drain the seepage of body fluids into those areas. There was a small air leak from one of my lungs and it was necessary to have a small amount of suction pressure applied to this until it sealed over.

As terrible as all this might sound, it was only when the chest tubes were eventually removed that there was considerable pain. Fortunately, this was temporary.

Some patients require the attachment of electrical pacing wires to the heart. These are brought out to the surface of the chest in case an electrical pacemaker is needed to keep the heart going. This the same type of pacemaker that is occasionally used after acute heart attacks. These are frequently also temporary. In other incidences, pacemakers are permanently implanted in persons who have very slow heart rates or pauses in the heart rate leading to blackout spells. This may occur even in the absence of a heart attack.

Fortunately, I escaped the need for these wires. My heart started beating on its own without the need for the usual application of an electrical shock.

Cognitive Function after Coronary Bypass Surgery

Duke is very much involved in the study of the effects of psychological and sociological factors on heart surgery. Consider the MOSS Study conducted by Judith Wheeler. MOSS is an acronym for Mediators of Social Support. This study was an attempt to evaluate by interview and questionnaire the role of religious beliefs, degree of self-esteem, depression, and availability of support from family and others. I take it that this study will evaluate prognosis and morbidity related to these factors. I am neither a psychologist nor a psychiatrist and so cannot evaluate the effectiveness of such data, but I did participate in the study to the best of my ability.

The role of coronary bypass surgery on cognitive function was of more interest, and seemed more practical, to me. Psychological testing was done for concentration, attention, and memory, both immediate and past, along with evaluation for depression and anxiety. Blood flow to the brain was measured during the operation. Those of us who participated were evaluated prior to heart surgery, after heart surgery but prior to hospital discharge, and again at six to seven weeks postoperative. I have been told that a six-month follow-up is also to be done. I felt that they were trying to determine how many brain cells I lost while on the heart-lung bypass machine during heart surgery.

The neuropsychological evaluations were conducted by Michelle Feldman under the direction of Dr. James Blumenthal, associate professor of Medical Psychology, along with Dr. J. G. Reves, professor and chair for the Department of Anesthesiology. Their results will be published when the study is complete. It is believed that the age of the patient and the duration of time one is on the bypass machine may influence the degree of loss of cognitive function. I had hoped that I would end up with a little better brain function after bypass surgery than I had before!

Bypass Surgery without a Blood Transfusion

My remaining two days in the hospital were uneventful. At no time did I have chest pain, except that derived from the surgery itself. I did not have shortness of breath. I felt some weakness, which I attributed to the fact that I was rather anemic. My red blood cell count declined from a normal one hundred percent before the operation to fifty-five percent after surgery. Some of this was probably a result of retention of extra fluid in my blood stream as a consequence of the use of the heart-lung machine. This is a common occurrence which is reversed with the use of a fluid pill (diuretic) during the first few days after surgery.

I did not receive a transfusion of blood during surgery. This is much comfort to almost everybody these days when there is such a fear for the transmission of AIDS, hepatitis, and other blood-borne infections. With modern testing, the odds for acquiring such an infection is extremely remote, but it is still comforting not to be exposed. At my office I am surprised by how much fear is noted in patients requiring blood transfusions. Some patients request a blood test for AIDS.

In elective surgery today, including coronary bypass operations, patients have what we call "auto-transfusions." That is, a patient donates his own blood in advance for the anticipated surgery. When the heart-lung bypass pump is used, blood is needed to prime the pump. In other words, a certain amount of blood is needed to initiate flow through the oxygenator, the heat exchanger, and the filter. In some instances there can be significant blood loss but this is not the general rule.

I know of a patient who was to undergo surgery for prostate cancer and donated two units of blood for his own use during surgery. The thinning of his blood caused him to develop chest pains of angina pectoris. Testing of his heart with an exercise electrocardiogram and catheterization revealed that coronary artery blockages were present. He underwent successful coronary bypass surgery and six weeks later had his prostate surgery.

Until recent years, many institutions, including Duke Medical Center, did not perform coronary bypass surgery on patients unless permitted to give blood products if it became necessary in the course of surgery. I have a patient who is a member of Jehovah's Witnesses, and who for religious reasons does not accept blood products. He traveled to the west coast for his surgery. More recently some institutions, including Duke, will perform such surgery under conditions of prior refusal of blood products. If in the course of my surgery there had been an indication for blood transfusion, I would not have opposed its use in the light of the accurate screening test today. Like others, I was pleased that the need did not arise.

The Hospital Discharge

It was early on Tuesday, the fifth day after my surgery, when Dr. Jones came on his morning rounds. He seemed to be in his usual pleasant mood. He listened to my heart and lungs. Then he carefully checked my sternal scar and the leg scar from which the saphenous vein had been taken. He seemed satisfied that all was well. He looked me straight in the eyes and said, "When would you like to go home? I usually let people go home when they think they are ready."

I know there was a grin on my face. I glanced out of the window and said, "It's mighty pretty outside. Looks to me like today would be a nice day for driving to Danville."

I knew Nez would be arriving from Betty's house in Raleigh very soon with expectations of my being discharged. I had already been up and about, walking with my portable monitor attached and had viewed the oscillograph at the nurses' station. I knew that my heart rhythm was perfect. I couldn't have felt better about the decision to be discharged.

Dr. Jones informed me that I would get an appointment card in the mail for follow-up with him in six weeks. He also gave me his hospital telephone extension number and his home telephone number in case I needed to reach him. I would have felt that this was a special privilege for me as a physician had I not known that other patients get the same instructions.

Dr. Ronald Lilly, the cardiac resident, came by to check on me and again examined my heart, lungs, and both of my incisions. I asked some questions about my use of blood thinners routinely used after coronary bypass surgery. He recalled that I was very intolerant to all forms of aspirin compounds. I mentioned the possibility of substituting dipyridamole (Persantine) for aspirin. He chose to defer this question to my cardiologist, Dr. Fetters, and agreed to ask her to come by.

I had other questions also. I wanted to talk with someone knowledgeable about my cholesterol panel. I felt I had been careful in restricting my dietary cholesterol and fatty acids. In the past I had considered drug therapy to try to lower my low-density cholesterol and raise my high-density fraction. All drugs for lowering cholesterol carry some risk. Otherwise, I would have already been on a medication. Now, knowing that I have extensive atherosclerotic disease in my coronary arteries, I felt that the risk of progressive cholesterol plaque formation far outweighs the risk of drug therapy. I wanted this opinion confirmed but Dr. Fetters did not get by to see me before I got away.

I left the hospital somewhat disappointed in regard to this aspect of my management. I now understand how those patients of ours may feel when they arrive at home and call the office to report that they were not properly told what medicines they should take or what their activity should be. Sometimes it has proved to be an oversight and sometimes it is a misunderstanding. Needless to say, I think I will try to be more cognizant of such matters in the future.

We had assistance in getting to the car and soon found our way toward Danville. We stopped in Hillsborough, N.C., at a pharmacy to have prescriptions filled. I appreciated the impact of the cost of medications more than ever before. I have been fortunate in requiring very few medications throughout my life. What I have needed has often been provided in the form of starter doses by a pharmaceutical representative at no cost to me. When I picked up the ticket for what seemed like a small amount of relatively inexpensive medication I thought to myself, "How in the world can poor people afford to be sick these days?" I have no insurance coverage for medications and this is true for most patients. I expressed this opinion to Nez's sympathetic ear.

When we arrived home I felt good about being there. There is a small lake in view of the house. There are five areas of grass around the lake which I prepared and regularly maintain to serve as golf greens. (See figure 8.) Trails between the greens are bordered with field stones, most of which I put there with my own hands. I partially credit this work for my good collateral circulation.

As soon as I dismounted from the car I walked around the lake with Nez sticking near by me. She later reported her marked anxiety about this walk. I had not known that she had witnessed a patient in the Stepdown Care have a cardiac arrest while walking following heart surgery.

I think that Westridge, as we call our country house, has been good for me and I expect it to continue to add to the years of my life. I wish every patient had the privilege of going home to a place they enjoy as much as I enjoy Westridge. Your home and grounds, including a garden or orchard, can be a source of excellent diversion and rehabilitation. I am fortunate in having acquired such a home site thirty-five years ago.

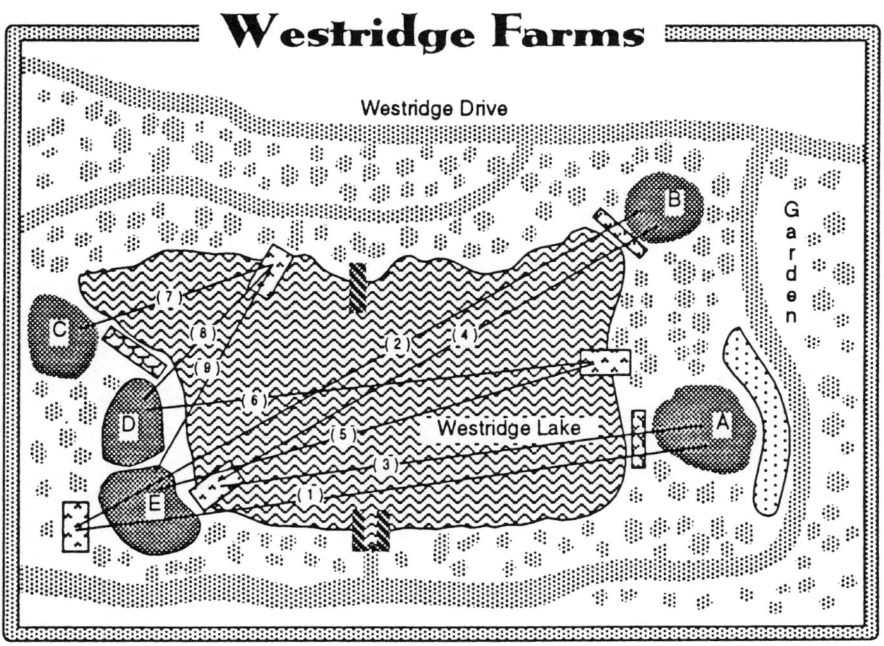

Figure 8. *Westridge Golf Course. The greens are marked alphabetically, with four greens being used twice for each nine-hole round.*

Protecting the New Grafts

"What can be done to protect my new grafts?" is a foremost question in the minds of those who have undergone a coronary artery bypass operation.

Blood Thinners

Aspirin is prescribed for virtually all persons who undergo coronary bypass surgery or balloon dilatation of the coronary arteries. It has been established that aspirin acts on the platelet cells to make them less sticky, making them less prone to create blood clots in the arteries that have just been repaired. This is one of the most effective and economical means of protecting the new grafts. Aspirin acts well in those who have had balloon dilatation or plaque removal by means of a rotating blade or laser.

There are a few individuals who are intolerant to aspirin. I happen to be one of those who is very sensitive to aspirin because of its stomach-irritating effect. Aspirin is a very effective medication for relief of minor aches and pains in muscles and joints. But I learned long ago that I could not take even small doses of aspirin without stomach discomfort. Recognizing its importance as a blood thinner, I agreed to try it again at Transylvania County Hospital. Almost immediately I developed considerable discomfort in my upper abdomen and had to omit it.

Dipyridamole (Persantine) and sulfinpyrazone (Anturane, sometimes used for gout) have an aspirin-like effect on platelets but they have not been well tested in large populations to establish their effectiveness, as has aspirin. I considered the use of Persantine in my own case and discussed this with my friend Dr. Robert Whalen, formerly chief of cardiology at Duke Medical Center. He felt its use was not sufficiently established to justify my taking it, but there are those who feel it is of value.

It should be remembered that acetaminophen (Tylenol), which is generally well tolerated, does not have the favorable effect on platelets as does aspirin.

Prevention of Cholesterol Plaque Disease

New grafts are subject to the same risk factors that lead to the development of cholesterol plaques in previously normal coronary arteries. It is therefore clear that good health habits are critical to the protection of the new grafts. If one has had the warning of a heart attack, or symptoms leading to catheterization and surgery on the coronary arteries, it becomes all the more important. Failure to identify and correct such factors will lead to the return of similar problems in the newly grafted arteries.

Control of Cholesterol

A diet low in cholesterol and saturated fatty acids is paramount in the management of the blood cholesterol level. My first interest in cholesterol began when I arrived at the University of Virginia in 1948. Dr. Ed Boyle was working on lipids (fats), using the ultracentrifuge. This instrument separated the blood fats based on their density. This was a big step forward in defining which of the blood fats was most harmful in causing diseases of the arteries.

At the time, the measurement of blood cholesterol was crude and inaccurate. I can remember when Ed and I would take blood from one patient and submit it to the clinical laboratory under five different names only to get a wide variety of results. Even today, with well-controlled laboratories that should come within five to ten percent accuracy, it is still important to verify results with a repeat test, before instituting medications.

All physicians who are interested in cholesterol problems will have copies of low cholesterol menus such as those prepared by the

American Heart Association. These will serve as helpful guides in choosing an appropriate diet. You should always obtain a lipid panel measured in a reliable laboratory. This will include total cholesterol, triglyceride, and high-density lipids (HDL). From these values, the low-density cholesterol (LDL), the harmful fraction, is calculated, and we can determine a risk factor for that given individual.

The HDL, or so-called good cholesterol fraction, is largely genetically determined but it can be improved through an exercise program, appropriate diet, and medications.

After a careful diet has been followed for three to four months, if the cholesterol continues high, one should at that point consider medication to further lower the cholesterol. Physicians generally determine the mathematical ratio between the HDL and the LDL to calculate the individual's risk. This is called the risk ratio. Your doctor or dietitian can explain this more fully.

The effectiveness of maintaining a low cholesterol level in the blood was established a few years ago in a classic study performed at the University of Southern California. The Cholesterol Lowering Atherosclerosis Study (CLAS) was a random study of 188 patients who had undergone coronary artery bypass surgery. The patients were divided into two groups, each of which was on a carefully controlled, low-fat, low-cholesterol diet. All were men between the ages of forty and fifty-nine, and were all nonsmokers. Each had undergone a coronary artery bypass operation and had angiograms done following the operation. One group took cholesterol-lowering medication while the other group received a placebo (a fake capsule with the appearance of the real medication).

At the beginning of the study each group had an average of 246 milligrams of total cholesterol. After two years of treatment, of the patients on diet and medication that lowered cholesterol only eighteen percent showed new evidence of grafts beginning closure. Of those who were on the placebo and diet without significant decrease in cholesterol, thirty percent showed evidence of beginning graft closure. These findings were confirmed by repeating the angiograms. Not only was there less closure developing in the new grafts, but less disease appeared in the native coronary arteries of some individuals. In some instances actual regression was demonstrated in the group taking medication.

Most experts in the field today are of the opinion that the total cholesterol in a person who has had bypass surgery should be well below the 200 milligram level. We would like this for the population as a whole. In all probability, any of the effective cholesterol-lowering medications available today will help protect grafts from re-occlusion. So far, all such medications have not been tested to the extent of two to four years. Your own physician can best determine which medications may be best for you.

Cholesterol-Lowering Medications

I won't discuss medications in great detail because this subject is too difficult to explain here. Drug therapy has to be individualized and should be given only under the direction of a competent physician. There are, however, some general observations that may be appropriate here.

Nicotinic acid use is apparently on the rise. Since this is the only medication available without prescription for the treatment of cholesterol problems, it is difficult to be sure of the frequency of its use. It is a medicine that does the right things to the blood fats. It lowers total cholesterol and triglycerides while raising the high-density lipids (HDL)—which is the good fraction. What may not be understood is the fact that enormous doses (2,000-3,000 milligrams per day) may be required to be effective. This is forty to sixty tablets of the regular fifty milligram strength, and may cause severe flushing of the skin. Undesirable flushing can often be abated by taking the tablets with food. An aspirin tablet taken shortly before the nicotinic acid is swallowed may also reduce flushing.

Long-acting nicotinic tablets have proven to be more toxic. While I have never seen a serious reaction to nicotinic acid that did not reverse itself on withdrawal of the medication, there have been incidents of fatal liver damage. I definitely feel that nicotinic acid treatment should be used only under the care of a physician who carefully monitors the necessary blood tests throughout treatment. It should be remembered that nicotinamide, which is also a member of the vitamin B complex group, does not have a favorable effect on cholesterol levels.

Bile sequestrant resins lower cholesterol by binding bile acids from the liver needed to absorb fats. They are generally available in a powder taken by mouth. The two resins available have trade names of Questran and Colestid. They have been proven effective in large trials, such as was done in the Lipid Research Clinics Program, conducted as early as 1984. These resins cause much gas and constipation, making patient acceptance poor. They may worsen the levels of triglycerides. They have a high rate of interaction with other drugs which heart patients often take. This demands special attention by the physician and patient.

Reductase inhibitors are the most recent additions to the medical management of cholesterol. Trade names are Mevacor, Pravacol, and Zocor. These drugs inhibit the manufacture of cholesterol by the liver through the blockage of HMG-CoA reductase, the enzyme necessary in cholesterol production. These medicines are easy to take and are generally well tolerated. Mevacor has been available longest and has been shown clearly effective in causing less progression and more regression of cholesterol deposits in blood vessels when taken in conjunction with an appropriate diet. It is likely that the other two drugs will be equally helpful when similar studies become available.

These medicines may cause serious liver damage or muscle pains (myalgia). Stomach upsets, headaches, and skin rashes are more common but not serious. Careful monitoring of blood studies is critical with the use of these medicines. The medications are more effective if given at bedtime since the liver produces most cholesterol between midnight and 3:00 a.m. The long-term consequences of these medications are not yet certain. Large doses in small animals have rarely caused liver cancer.

Gemfibrozil (Lopid) is effective in reducing triglycerides and raising HDL, both of which are desirable effects. There is less effect on the

LDL cholesterol than some other cholesterol-lowering medications. In a large Helsinki test done a few years ago, it proved effective primarily in those persons who had lower levels of HDL.

Probucol (Lorelco) is said to work as an antioxidant medication. (Oxidation tends to cause LDL cholesterol to exert its harmful effect.) It tends to lower HDL cholesterol along with LDL. The lowering of HDL, since this is the "good fraction," is of uncertain significance but has led to concern.

Fish oils, which are present in cold-water fish and commercially available in capsules, contain highly unsaturated omega-3 fatty acids. These can lower triglycerides and slightly lower (or elevate) low-density cholesterol. In a two-year study of men who have had heart attacks, they have been shown to lower death rates by twenty-nine percent.

Combinations of medications are sometimes used when single drug therapy is ineffective. Even though more effective, adverse reactions are greatly enhanced; therefore, drug combinations should be administered only under careful observation by a competent physician.

There are a number of medications and substances known as antioxidants. They are helpful in the prevention of oxidation of cholesterol, the process that causes fats to become rancid. Their ability to prevent coronary heart disease, either with or without influencing cholesterol levels, is not as well established as the medications we have discussed. Along with Probucol, mentioned above, there are a number of nonprescription medicines that act as antioxidants. Among these are vitamin C, vitamin E, vitamin A, and certain trace metals, such as zinc. The Harvard Physician's Health Study, in which I volunteered to participate, evaluated beta-carotene (a precursor of vitamin A). The results showed a significant improvement in the prevention of heart attacks and strokes in those physicians getting beta-carotene. Other substances, such as garlic, will require more closely controlled evaluation. Though promising, the study on the use of walnuts for the lowering of cholesterol was limited to a very small group of men and for a very short duration. It is unsure what the long-range effects may be on a larger group. It has not been established that walnuts are more effective than other nuts. All nuts are high in calories and make weight control more difficult.

Since my bypass operation, I have taken daily vitamin A, C, E, zinc, and a multivitamin with minerals. Nez has recommended this for a long time but I have been compliant only since my surgery. The main factor in using the antioxidant agents is the fact that their use is very safe, which cannot be said for the prescription medications, unless they are carefully monitored.

Cigarettes

Cigarette smoking and elevated cholesterol levels constitute by far the two greatest hazards to the coronary artery circulation of the heart. All forms of tobacco, whether in cigarettes (with or without filters), cigars, or pipes, or as tobacco with reduced nicotine—all carry a hazard. This is true not only for the heart but for all blood vessels. Secondhand smoke is hazardous as well. Other members of the household should be aware of this.

Tobacco smoking has recently been shown to cause significant elevations in blood pressure. The pressure elevation may subside in less than an hour after the cigarette is smoked, hence, the effect may not be detected in the physician's office, where smoking is prohibited. Proof of the effect of smoking on blood pressure has been best established using a continuous (ambulatory) monitor which checks readings throughout the entire twenty-four hour period. Spikes in elevated pressures often correlate with the time of smoking.

Programs to aid in quitting smoking are available, including nicotine in the form of chewing gum and the transdermal nicotine patch applied to the skin. These are available by prescription and can be an aid to the individual who is addicted but is serious about quitting. Less accepted by the medical profession are techniques such as hypnosis and acupuncture. All the aids used in stopping smoking are relatively expensive, but each will prove to be economical in the long run, if effective.

Hypertension

High blood pressure adds stress to the heart and blood vessels, including the coronary arteries. It is true that hypertension is a greater risk in producing strokes than it is in causing coronary heart attacks. It can cause enlargement and weakness of the heart, however, which leads to failure of the heart muscle to function adequately. It is important that blood pressure be effectively controlled, and a variety of medications can assist in the effort. Some high blood pressure medications may tend to elevate the blood cholesterol level, but in most instances this effect is a transient one. The cholesterol should be monitored and managed appropriately in the presence of any antihypertensive medication.

Some blood pressure medications have added benefits on the heart. Some of the beta-blocker group of medicines have been shown to decrease the probability of subsequent heart attacks, especially during the first year after an initial attack. Some benefit may be derived by administering drugs such as atenolol (Tenormin®) and metoprolol (Lopressor®) intravenously at the first sign of a heart attack resulting in improved prognosis.

The ACE-inhibitor drugs lower blood pressure, at least in part, by blocking the angiotensin-converting enzyme, which helps raise blood pressure. These same medicines are being proved to prolong life in patients who have weakened hearts due to coronary artery disease. This growing group of medicines include captopril (Capoten®), enalapril (Vasotec®), fosinopril (Monopril®), lisinopril (Prinivil®, Zestril®), and ramipril (Altace™).

A host of other medicines are available for lowering blood pressure.

Obesity

Being overweight is a risk factor for the heart, although perhaps not as great as those listed above. Being overweight tends to aggravate other conditions, such as diabetes mellitus, hypertension, and high cholesterol, all of which are risk factors in themselves. It is important for you to try to maintain a constant weight within the limits of normal for your height.

Exercise

An exercise program should be instituted immediately upon discharge from the hospital following bypass surgery. The type and degree of exercise should be prescribed by your physician. If you have suffered a heart attack with some damage to the heart muscle, your exercise program will have to be much more graduated. If your heart function is diminished, as demonstrated by a low ejection fraction at the time of your catheterization, then the proper degree of exercise likewise will be limited.

Older patients, especially those who have reached beyond the sixth or seventh decade, may have associated nonheart problems, such as arthritis, which may restrict the type and degree of activity possible. Fortunately for me, I had a good ejection fraction (sixty-five percent), and have no other limiting disabilities (except arthritis in the neck) to keep me from doing a full exercise program. For some of us, exercising can be somewhat boring. I much prefer to do my exercise outside where I can jog or maintain a garden, grass, and shrubs. During cold and otherwise inclement weather, facilities for inside exercise should be available. I prefer a stationary bicycle. I find that using the stationary bicycle while watching television can be far less boring. If one begins exercise at the onset of the evening news and continues this until the conclusion of the program, it serves both as a diversion and a timer.

Exercises that I enjoy most, such as digging, raking, pruning, and gardening, are less desirable because they do not enable one to maintain an increased heart rate for a period of time. Playing golf while walking and carrying your own bag can provide a certain amount of pleasure and diversion. Those who have strong hearts and good endurance may get a great deal of satisfaction out of competitive physical sports like tennis.

To participate in vigorous activity, the treadmill stress test should serve as a guide for your physician to prescribe an appropriate exercise program. I have learned that it is better to try to tailor an exercise program to a patient's ability and interest than to waste time discussing a program that the patient will not follow. For those who are proven to be satisfactory candidates, optimal benefits are achieved from twenty minutes of vigorous exercise three or four times per week.

Alcohol and the Heart

The role of a couple of ounces of alcohol a day in the prevention of coronary heart disease is still a controversial one. I can remember as far back as medical school when one of my professors used to advocate, "He who takes a daily drink before the age of fifty is foolish, and he who does not take a daily drink after the age of fifty is likewise foolish."

There has been some scientific indication that one and one-half to two ounces of alcohol a day may favorably influence the level of HDL (the good fraction) of cholesterol in the blood. There are at least three fractions of HDL, and there is still some controversy as to whether the fraction of the HDL that increases with alcohol is the same fraction that helps prevent coronary artery disease. Since I have not taken alcoholic beverages on any regular basis, I have no way of knowing whether I have denied myself benefit or not.

When the discussion of the merits of alcohol is mentioned, I am reminded of an anecdote one of my late colleagues used to tell. He was lecturing an alcoholic on the evils of alcohol, and how it might kill him, when he got this response: "I tell you, Doc, I know a whole lot more old drunks than I do old doctors." I think the evidence is not all in. Certainly there are potential harmful effects from alcohol that might outweigh any benefits that may be seen on the coronary arteries.

It is important to remember that excessive use of alcohol can lead to certain cardiovascular disorders.

(1) Hypertension is clearly caused by alcohol in some individuals. I have persuaded a number of persons to give up alcohol and demonstrated that their blood pressures are significantly improved, and may even become normal.

(2) Myocarditis is a form of muscle degeneration of the heart that is seen on occasion in chronic alcoholics. I have seen a few such persons become very ill due to weakness of the heart. Outlook is poor, for, in my experience, medical treatment is generally futile. Heart transplantation may prove the only effective management when heart damage is advanced.

There are many hazards of alcohol abuse that will not be discussed here. Suffice it to say that the liver damage, pancreas damage, brain injury, and stomach ulcers are all serious and well-documented complications of alcohol excess. Motor vehicle accidents, domestic violence, and economic disaster are problems well recognized as being associated with alcohol abuse.

The use of one to two ounces of wine daily has recently created widespread interest because of a report from France late in 1992 that appeared in the journal *The Lancet*. There was significant newspaper and television coverage of the finding that the French, who have a rather high intake of cholesterol and saturated fats in their diets, have a low incidence of coronary heart disease. While it has been previously reported that two ounces of wine, and perhaps other alcoholic beverages in equivalent amounts, have favorable effects on the HDL (good fraction), this study emphasizes the importance of wine on the blood clotting mechanism. The blood platelets, which influence the clotting of blood, have less reactivity in those persons who consume a small amount of wine daily. This would suggest that the mechanism is similar to what is found in those who take an aspirin daily. There is evidence that more than two ounces of alcohol, especially in the form of binge or heavy weekend drinking, may actually increase the chances of developing coronary heart disease.

It seems clear that the role of alcohol in helping or harming the heart requires further careful study.

The Sensuous Heart

Why is it that every television talk show, every sitcom, and every newsstand magazine talks about sex, but when you have a serious problem with the heart, doctors and nurses become mute on the subject? No doubt there should be an association between the recommendation of abstinence of sex and the degree of heart damage and the lapse of time since surgery. The wounds have to undergo a certain amount of healing so as to not be painful. Persons who have suffered recent heart attacks will need to abstain from sex for three to six weeks. Those who have surgery without associated heart damage will be managed differently. They can participate as soon as their wounds are no longer painful. Patients who have a catheterization alone are limited until there is no threat of bleeding, which is usually only a day or two.

There are the physical factors and psychological factors. The amount of exertion required for sex is about the same as climbing two flights of stairs. There is evidence that moderate exercise enhances an active sex life at all ages. If this is true in healthy persons, I see no reason for believing it is not so in those who have had heart problems including those who have had heart surgery.

Vigorous exercise, such as competitive long-distance running, may cause low sperm counts in men and disturbed ovulation in women. These effects are related to lower sex harmones; testosterone in men, and estrogen in women. Fewer studies have been done in women than in men. More open discussions about sexual activity after heart attacks and heart surgery are certainly appropriate and can allay many unnecessary fears. It is a known fact that extramarital sex is more hazardous in the presence of heart disease, but I doubt if this is frequently a problem following cardiac surgery.

I have drawn a few conclusions about this complex subject in heart patients. Maybe the important factor is hormones! When the sex hormone level reaches a certain point, it probably means that the heart is also about ready. I cannot definitely support all of the above suggestions, but then there are not many double-blind, scientifically designed studies to give us concise answers on this subject. My conclusion is that a repaired heart is still compatible with good sex!

There are a number of medications prescribed for the heart and high blood pressure that may cause relative impotence. You may need to inquire about this possibility. In all likelihood, the doctor will not bring this up. Often there is another medication that may be equally as effective and that may result in no adverse effect on sexual function.

Genes May Be Important

Genetic factors play an important role in a variety of heart diseases. Family clusters of coronary heart disease are evident. Heart attacks in identical twins show a greater degree of concordance than we see in fraternal twins. In other words, if one identical twin has coronary heart disease the incidence of the same heart disease is greater in the identical sibling than it would be in a fraternal twin sibling. Families with consistently high cholesterol levels (familial hypercholesterolemia) and families with high triglycerides (familial hypertriglyceridemia) are at a distinctly higher risk for early coronary heart disease. Those families who have lower levels of high density cholesterol (HDL, the good fraction) are also at increased risk.

My first direct contact with familial hypercholesterolemia (FH) came about four decades ago, when I learned that a medical colleague had the disorder. He was an obstetrician. He delivered our last three children and I helped with the management of his heart problem. In spite of an effort to restrict his dietary cholesterol, his blood levels remained between 350 and 600 milligrams. He had first shown evidence of heart trouble in the form of angina pectoris at the age of twenty-eight years. He suffered a full-blown heart attack (myocardial infarction) at the age of forty-one. During his fifty-fourth year he had a fatal heart attack while playing golf. At the time of his death he was the longest surviving member of his immediate family. His father died at forty. One brother died at thirty-four and another at forty. Subsequently, a son has died at forty-nine years after having had a heart attack at forty. With today's modern medications, outlook for improved longevity is significantly greater. The use of multiple medications is sometimes necessary.

The presence of low HDL appears to be a factor in my own family's tendency to arteriosclerotic disease, especially coronary heart disease. Observe in the table (see figure 9) that all four of my siblings have abnormally low or borderline low levels of HDL, as I have. The triglycerides are nearly always normal and in every incidence except one (Aaron) total cholesterol and LDL are within normal limits.

Because of its prevalence in the general population, the most significant familial disorder associated with abnormal cholesterol finding is diabetes mellitus. In diabetes, especially if poorly controlled, there is a high incidence of cholesterol problems. There is an associated high incidence of coronary heart disease. There is also a high incidence of other arteriosclerotic disorders such as carotid artery blockage, kidney artery blockage and strokes.

To further amplify the complexity of genetic factors in cholesterol metabolism, there was an interesting article in the *New England Journal of Medicine* in 1991. Much attention was given to the report of an eighty-eight-year-old man who had consumed twenty-five eggs daily for a period of more than fifteen years. The accuracy of his compulsive behavior was confirmed by his physician and friends. His lipid profile, including total cholesterol, triglycerides, and high-density cholesterol were entirely normal. He had no signs of significant blood vessel disease. Special studies revealed that he had poor cholesterol absorption from the intestinal tract along with other factors that interfered with cholesterol production.

I have occasionally encountered patients who have consumed large amounts of cholesterol (not to the extent of twenty-five eggs per day) who have maintained normal lipid levels. This situation is rare. Perhaps some day we will select such individuals and permit them to consume a diet without regard to their fat intake. In the meantime, I feel I have an obligation to continue to point out the potential hazards of excessive dietary cholesterol.

Gene therapy for some cardiovascular diseases is rapidly developing in the laboratory and will soon enter clinical trials. It will likely be many years before this therapy can be adapted to the management of coronary heart disease, but it does hold hope for the

SUMMARY OF AUTHOR'S FAMILY CHOLESTEROL VALUES

	Normal Values	Author	Sidney	Maston	Duncan	Aaron
Age at Onset of Attack*		68	54	61	71	64
Current Age		68	85	75	73	71
Total Cholesterol	(140-199)	190	177	165	160	245
Triglycerides	(30-190)	150	143	228	292	108
LDL(Bad)	(60-160)	122	116	146	77	183
HDL(Good)	(30-80)	30	32	28	25	40
Risk Ratio TC/HDL	(< 5.1)	6.3	5.8	5.6	6.4	6.1

*All attacks have been coronary artery disease except Aaron. His was carotid artery blockage with surgery. Note the consistently low HDL values leading to a high TC/HDL ratio.

Figure 9. *Summary of the author's family cholesterol values.*

future. Meanwhile, it is important for us to identify the genetic predisposition to coronary heart disease in order that one can more rigidly apply management to correct other risk factors. It becomes all the more important for a genetically predisposed individual to follow a low-cholesterol, low-saturated-fatty-acid diet, to abstain from cigarette smoking, to avoid obesity, and to correct hypertension. Had I been more alert to the presence of low HDL in my family, perhaps measures could have been taken to improve this risk factor, particularly the administration of medications that tend to improve its level. I must confess that I did not investigate the lipid patterns of my brothers until I suffered my own attack.

It is only sensible to keep alert to the discovery of other cholesterol fractions that may have an influence of coronary artery disease. I suspect that during the course of the next decade, we will hear more about such factors as LPa and apoE. They are factors that are genetically determined. These risk factors are known in the laboratory today just as HDL was a decade ago. You are likely to hear more about these and other factors in the future.

Just a few years ago, I attended a patient who was in his late sixties, but had undergone coronary bypass surgery, had an aneurysm of the aorta removed, and had a mild stroke. Circulation in his feet and legs was extremely poor. He had had cholesterol plaques removed from both of his carotid arteries. His total cholesterol values ranged around 150 to 160 with normal triglycerides. Knowledge about HDL was relatively new, and when we measured his, we found it to be only twelve (preferred normal values are above forty milligrams). Prior to the discovery of the HDL fraction, the cause of his extensive blood vessel disease would have been obscure. Additional new risk factors among the blood fats (lipids) are likely to be uncovered in the years ahead.

Coronary Artery Surgery of the Future

It is interesting to speculate about the future of coronary artery surgery. The number of women undergoing coronary artery bypass (CAB) surgery is increasing significantly. It is estimated that there are more than 300,000 CAB operations being done each year. There is nearly an equal number of coronary balloon dilatations done on an annual basis, and this number seems to be growing. As I have commented before, approximately one-third of those undergoing this procedure will require repeat dilatations.

Also, procedures for removing the cholesterol plaques with a rotating blade as well as removing them with the laser beam are becoming increasingly popular. The group at Cleveland Clinic has randomized a series of patients in two categories. Those who got direct cholesterol plaque removal had fifteen percent lower return of blockage at six months than those who had dilatation with the balloon.

It appears that bypass surgery and balloon angioplasty are clearly here to stay. Other procedures may come to the forefront. Dr. Robert Califf, who arranged my helicopter transfer to Duke Medical Center, is very much involved in these studies. There will, of course, continue to be refinements to make the procedures safer and increasingly more effective.

Over the course of the next decade we may see coronary angiograms done with the catheter being replaced by a noninvasive technique utilizing ultrasound, which is currently being used to study larger arteries. Also, there are recent reports of the use of magnetic resonance imaging (MRI) to visualize blockages in the coronary arteries. A recent addition to coronary artery evaluation is the use of

MRI to find calcium deposits in the vessel walls. Where calcium is found arterioslerosis is likely to be present. Those with excess calcium on the screening test may deserve further study, such as catheterization. The preliminary results of MRI appear favorable. This technique would also eliminate the use of catheters and needles, something that would be welcome by most of us.

In an era when there in so much concern over the increasing cost of health care, one wonders what restrictions on these invasive procedures will develop. Heart transplants are becoming more prevalent. As studies uncover improved means to avoid tissue rejection, a greater number of transplants will be performed, if adequate donors become available. The cost of these procedures is astronomical. Currently, the all-inclusive costs (hospital, nursing care, anesthesia, and professional charges) for these high-tech and highly skilled procedures are approximately as follows: catheterization, $4,000; balloon angioplasty, $6,000; coronary artery bypass operation, $55,000; heart transplant, $95,000. These costs vary significantly, based on the need, for example, for helicopter transport, the general health of the patient, and potential complications.

Who will pay for these expensive procedures? What about those persons who have not reached Medicare age and are not insured? There will be a growing demand on Medicare and Medicaid at a time when there is a great effort under way to put a cap on the cost of medical care.

Will there be restrictions based on age? When the first bypass procedures were done, it was felt that persons over the age of fifty-five to sixty should not be considered as candidates for the operation. Our concept has undergone quite a change. Take a friend and patient of mine, for example, who is in his eighty-first year. He came to see me about a month prior to my own surgery and reported that he was having some discomfort in his chest as he walked up grade to the greens on the golf course. We did a treadmill stress test that was clearly abnormal. I had attended his father, who lived to the age of 101, and the son fully expects to live just as long. When a short period of medical treatment was not fully effective, he opted right away to have a catheterization. He chose to go to Duke Medical Center where Dr. Peter did his catheterization, and a successful coronary artery bypass operation was done by Dr. Robert Jones. In the course of his evaluation of the coronary arteries, it was discovered that he had an aneurysm (a dangerous ballooning) of his aorta. To repair this aneurysm was a more serious operation than the coronary bypass procedure. Approximately four weeks after his coronary artery bypass an operative repair of the aneurysm was done and ten days following his second surgery he was attending church and other meetings. He tells me he is now anxiously awaiting permission to get back on the golf course.

I am a firm believer that individuals should be considered by their biological age (that is, the state of their health) rather than their chronological age (the number of birthdays) and should be managed accordingly. I am not sure that Medicare, Medicaid, and other third party agencies can adequately make such decisions.

Duke University Medical Center has just reported its results on eighty-six octogenarians and nonagenarians (age eighty to ninety-three) who have undergone coronary artery surgery. The results were remarkably good. This very elder group remained in the hospital only ten days (the average is seven for those younger). Eighty-eight percent returned home and the twelve percent who went to nursing homes did so only because of lack of assistance at home.

Patients on kidney dialysis machines have previously been regarded as unsuitable for coronary artery bypass surgery. A group of twenty-one persons on dialysis has had such surgery at Duke Medical Center with a death rate of only nine percent. The five-year survival was sixty percent in this group.

Persons with other significant illnesses, such as diabetes and chronic lung disease, are no longer being denied the benefits of the operation. As the government commands more and more control over the practice of medicine, the greater the philosophic and economic problems become. Someone, I hope someone well qualified will make the serious decisions about where our health dollars will be spent.

Should invasive testing and invasive treatments always be carried out? When my oldest brother had his first evidence of coronary disease thirty-one years ago we were not doing catherizations. Balloon angioplasty and coronary bypass surgery had hardly reached the stage of imagination. While today my brother is in poor cardiovascular health, there are those who have had invasive therapy who have done less well. I could say the same about my second-oldest brother, who had his heart attack in 1979, and has been very productive on medical treatment without ever having been catheterized.

In 1968, I treated a thirty-six-year-old accountant in our emergency department with severe chest pain which appeared abruptly while he was preparing for a fishing trip. He was weak and sweating and his electrocardiogram showed a blood clot on the back surface of his heart. At that time we had no continuous heart monitoring system in the emergency department, but continuous recording of his electrocardiogram showed what we call a complete heart block. There was no conduction of impulses from the small chambers of his heart to the lower ventricles. He had extremely long pauses in his heart beat lasting up to seven to nine seconds. Today, an immediate pacemaker would have been inserted by way of a catheter into his heart to stimulate a regular normal rate. At that time we were able only to give him medication (atropine) which successfully enhanced the heart rate. After four weeks in the hospital, which was the usual period of time in those days, he was discharged doing well. He continues to do well twenty-five years later in spite of the fact that we did not have the modern technology that we would use today. I am certainly happy modern technology was available for my treatment and for others today. But we forget patients often did well prior to the days of sophisticated measures.

Today, patients and their families expect more from modern technology than is available. We are under greater pressure to apply the modern techniques, else we might be held liable.

Good health habits with the avoidance of risk factors will help avert the development of coronary heart disease but we all know that the aging process eventually catches up. There are also those who have genetic factors such as inherited cholesterol disorders, diabetes, or low thyroid states that predispose them to coronary heart disease. We will always have to deal with such conditions even when there are no other preventable risk factors involved.

Nothing Good Comes Cheap

Having been home now for six weeks, and the bills having all (I hope) arrived, there are some suggestions that I have to make. If you are planning to have coronary bypass surgery, you must be sure to be either (1) independently wealthy or (2) to be sixty-five or older so that your Medicare will rescue you, and have an appropriate supplement to help with what your Medicare does not cover.

Further suggestions are as follows: Make sure that you are near a medical center that does heart surgery when you have your attack of chest pain. If it produces serious injury to your heart or produces irregularity of your heartbeat, you may need to be transferred in a hurry. The helicopter is a great device, but it was designed for the critically ill who can afford it. Keep in mind the takeoff fee is $1,500 and then you are charged by the mile. The flight mileage fee for me, I figure, was about $150 a mile. There was the cost of transport oxygen, intravenous fluids, testing of oxygen levels, and two well-trained coronary care nurses plus the pilot. It is definitely preferable to have your attack close to the coronary care unit or operating room. I have concluded that if I do another high-wire rope walk it will be on the grounds of a medical center.

I understand better than most patients why certain medications should be quite expensive. A sleeping pill purchased on prescription at a drugstore might be fifty cents each; but if it is in a hospital where it is dispensed by a druggist, transported to the nursing unit, administered by a well-trained coronary care nurse, and charted on the record by an experienced secretary, might well cost $7.65, as mine did. I am at a bit of a loss, however, as to why a Tylenol tablet cost only $3.15 when a half-strength chewable baby aspirin cost $5.55.

It all adds up to a little more than $7,000 a day, so long as you do not consider the cost of your operating surgeon, your catheterization expert and your anesthesiologist. If you are fortunate enough to come out feeling in good health and prepared to resume normal activity after your postoperative recovery, then you feel it has all been quite worthwhile. As Nez said, as we were leaving Transylvania County hospital, "What good is money if you are not here to spend it?"

Chest Pain Is No Respector of Gender

Nez had been having some discomfort with her chest for three months. In August 1992, she was involved in a taxicab accident in Chicago, and sustained a rib fracture, which had continued to annoy her. Then, the week I arrived home, she slipped on the ice on the deck at the house and fractured her right hand. There was also the possibility that this fall might have further aggravated her chest pain. For about four weeks, she had on occasion felt that she was having some increased shortness of breath and tightness in her chest on exertion. An electrocardiogram showed the presence of a left bundle branch block, that had not been present on her previous tracing, about five years earlier.

The finding of a conduction abnormality on the electrocardiogram, as was demonstrated with the bundle branch block, is often non-specific. It eliminates the electrocardiogram as an important tool in further studying the heart in a noninvasive fashion. I sought the advice of our cardiologist, who concurred in my feelings that we would probably have to do a cardiac catheterization in order to establish the significance of these symptoms and findings. Dr. Robert Peter at Duke Medical Center was consulted. He was the cardiologist who had done my catheterization just seven weeks before. He agreed with our conclusion that a catheterization would be needed.

When we arrived at Duke the cath lab nurse laughingly told us, "If Mrs. Gaddy has coronary artery surgery so soon after yours, we will have to report this in the *New England Journal of Medicine*."

We physicians have been accused of being neglectful about evaluating women for heart disease. I think this is a legitimate accusation.

There are reasons why we are more hesitant in suspecting the diagnosis in women than in men. First of all, women are much less prone to develop coronary heart disease before the menopausal years. We may be inclined to forget that following menopause, statistics on women with heart disease rapidly approaches that of men. Another problem is the fact that in women, the electrocardiogram, especially done during treadmill exercise, is far less specific than it is in men. The test does become more specific if we do a so-called Thallium scan. We inject a small amount of radioactive Thallium material into the vein near the conclusion of exercise and then proceed with testing. This is done in the X-ray department with an updated Geiger counter and scanner.

Women, as a whole, do not respond as well to coronary bypass surgery or to balloon angioplasty as do men. This is probably another important reason why more aggressive diagnostic tests are not done in females. I think cardiologists today are rethinking our position about women and are being more aggressive about evaluating their chest pains.

Why women have a later-in-life onset of heart disease as compared to men is uncertain. It has been suspected that there must be a relationship to the female hormone estrogen. The natural withdrawal of estrogen leading to menopause seems to coincide with the accelerated incidence of coronary heart disease in women. This has been a long-standing observation. Further support for this likely association is the more recent finding that women who take synthetic estrogen, such as Premarin, following menopause have a significant reduction in the incidence of heart attacks. The use of female hormones is not completely without risks. Cancer of the uterus appears in a slight but definite increase. The need for regular Pap smears is important. When another sex hormone (progesterone) is given in conjunction with estrogen there seems to be less risk of uterine cancer, but this may tend to counter the favorable effect on the heart. Other studies have not supported such an unfavorable effect. On the contrary, well-controlled studies recently reported indicate the combined hormones may produce an even better effect on the cholesterol panel. The role of female hormones in the development of breast cancer is less certain, but are held in suspect by many while others think the evidence is insufficient for a conclusion.

Now, it should be clear why the practice of medicine is such a challenge, and sometimes such a frustration. It should be no surprise that patients are often given opposing opinions on a given subject. We are still in search of many answers.

Arrangements were made for us to arrive at Duke Medical Center early the following day. We arrived at the Medical Center at 7:00 a.m. and began the preliminaries of paper work and laboratory tests to establish normal tendency for her blood to clot. Then we waited five hours for our turn to enter the catheterization laboratory.

Nez enjoys relating the interview that she had with the physician's assistant who came to describe the catheterization procedure to her. After relating some of the technicalities of the procedure, she added, "I must also tell you that this, being a surgical procedure, involves some risk. You might have a blood clot move to your lungs, or to your brain producing a stroke, and there is a chance that you might die from the procedure."

Since I knew that statistically there was only one fatality in approximately 2,500 procedures, I felt that I could further reassure her and point out that the procedure was probably less of a hazard than going to the mailbox for the newspaper, especially if there was a little ice on the deck!

When Nez was taken to the cath lab, this time it was my turn to suffer the anxiety of waiting for results, wondering what I would do should she have to undergo coronary bypass surgery. It was hard for me to believe she could have serious trouble. Nez had good health habits. She never had a high-cholesterol diet, she never smoked, she never had high blood pressure. Her family history for heart disease was much more favorable than mine. Her father died early of an accident and although her mother had a heart attack at age seventy-five she lived until ninety without further trouble with her heart. As for stress, my type A personality must be more stressful to her than her type B personality is for me. She's always been the greatest when it came to being calm, patient, and understanding.

Fortunately, her heart function, as measured by the ejection fraction, was good, and the coronary arteries appeared quite healthy. The nature of her chest discomfort is still not clear. Whether it was spasm in the coronary arteries rather than a blockage due to cholesterol (atherosclerosis) is not certain. The hurting may have originated outside the heart, such as in the ribs or muscles, and may have been due to her previous injuries. Sometimes such hurting can originate from the esophagus (gullet) or gall bladder disease. If hurting persists, such possibilities require investigation.

It was a great relief to find Nez's coronary blood vessels to be healthy. As noted earlier, up to thirty percent of catheterizations done each year for chest pain suspected of being due to heart disease will result in normal angiograms.

Nez found the catheterization procedure to be a very easy one, as had I. Women are generally somewhat more stoic than men. At least women say so, and I have to agree from my own observation and experience. She described the procedure as being easier than some trips to the dental office, but then not all dentists are the same.

After four hours of pressure to the groin area she was permitted to walk. There being no indication of bleeding, we were told she could be discharged and go home. One-day surgery units for heart catheterization have proven safe and represent quite a change from the past. It is a move in the direction of economy for medical care.

Betty and Steve remained with us throughout the day, offering their support. They encouraged us to stay in the Chapel Hill-Raleigh area for the night, but we elected to return to Westridge. It was then my responsibility to see that she was without physical activity for two days. I succeeded.

A Cruise for Recovery

Shortly after arriving home from the hospital, I felt the urge to do something different. We were having many calls and visits by friends, which was nice, but I wanted to get away for a while. By chance at the Rotary Club, I met a friend who operates a travel agency, and asked him what was available for cruises at that time. He assured me that there had never been better bargains in cruises. He gave me information to prove that he was absolutely correct.

On the following day I started walking from the house to get the morning newspaper about 150 yards away. Nez insisted that I should not do that because there were wet leaves in the driveway and I might slip and fall. She hurriedly grabbed her shoes, pulled them on and started down from the deck when she stepped on an icy area, falling and fracturing her right wrist. Her cast was in place for a period of six weeks. With this incident, I felt we needed the cruise more than ever. Since Nez was doing so much for me and now had only a left hand to do it with, we needed a place where our meals and entertainment would be provided without effort on our part.

We flew out of Raleigh-Durham Airport on Monday, November 16. It was the first and only time that I had the occasion to take advantage of an airport's facilities for the handicapped. Frankly, I prefer to do it all on my own, but in this instance, there was no option. By midday we had arrived at San Juan, Puerto Rico.

We boarded the S.S. *Amerikanis*, an older vessel that had been refurbished and was extraordinarily clean and well staffed.

The ship's food was excellent for all five daily meals, making it horribly difficult on one who feels that he should be even more restricted in his calories and cholesterol foods than ever before. It was a good opportunity to exercise self-discipline because heart-healthy food was available. The temptation was great to take many forbidden foods.

It was a pleasure to meet the ship's captain, Captain I. Papanikolaou. This was a familiar name to me because it was Dr. Papanikolaou who made famous the Pap test that has been so effective in screening for female cancer of the cervix and uterus.

At our table was a retired submarine officer. He liked to talk about his excellent health and attributed it to taking three cloves of fresh garlic, which he brought to the table wrapped in a napkin each evening at dinner. He was not able to explain the mechanism by which the garlic was so effective in keeping him healthy. Nez suggested that he was protected from infectious diseases because his garlic breath kept everyone else at a distance. There are those who believe that garlic, acting as an antioxidant, can be useful in helping prevent coronary heart disease. Since I was only four weeks past my coronary artery bypass surgery, heart disease was a common subject at the dinner hour.

Activities aboard the ship were generally interesting, but for someone who likes to be active, it was somewhat distressing to stay aboard and spend a few minutes in the swimming pool on the deck while others were going on tours for snorkeling and scuba diving. I could not participate in volleyball, a basketball shooting tournament and certainly with my four weeks' old sternal splitting scar, did not care about participating in trap shooting.

One evening after I had been swimming in the pool, a gentleman stopped me to ask, "Did you have your operation at Cleveland Clinic?"

I said, "No, I had mine at Duke University Medical Center," and wondered why he asked.

He said, "Well, your scar looks just like mine."

Never before had I considered that a surgical scar might be distinctive for a given institution, like a trademark!

During the afternoon lull in excitement, if you did not take a shore cruise, you were invited to play bridge or participate in ballroom dance classes.

Each evening there was worthwhile entertainment and there was always the opportunity to make a contribution to the slot machines or to play Jackpot Bingo.

After eight days and seven port calls we were ready for disembarkation and transportation back to the San Juan Airport.

We arrived back at Raleigh/Durham and were met by Steve and Betty. We were assisted with our luggage and invited to remain in Chapel Hill or Raleigh for the night. We chose to make our way back to Danville and to Westridge. We arrived home refreshed and ready to pick up our rehabilitation where we had left off. The cruise was a source of diversion from what we had undergone through the preceding four weeks. It allowed activity at the prescribed level and permitted an appropriate menu for one to exercise will power in dieting. It allowed another week to move closer to resuming the activities of normal daily living.

I can recommend a cruise for recovery.

Resuming Life Again

The anniversary of the eighth week after surgery was a gratifying one. I returned for my treadmill examination and found that my resting electrocardiogram was now entirely normal. You couldn't prove from the EKG that a heart problem had ever existed. The treadmill test was quite difficult and very tiresome. My body muscles were out of condition due to limited activity during the previous two months. It is true that I had been recently doing some fast walking and a small amount of jogging, but nothing like my normal activity.

We elected to do the treadmill test that utilizes the Bruce protocol, as I described in an earlier chapter. I began to fatigue relatively early, but there was no discomfort in my chest and I was not particularly short of breath, so I chose to continue exercise. As we proceeded, I was asked if I wanted to abort the test, but I continued throughout the twelve-minute protocol. I was watching the monitor throughout and I was fully aware of the fact that the tracing was looking good without changes of limited circulation, and there were no irregular beats. I wanted to complete the entire protocol since this would make it much more helpful for future comparisons.

As we began the treadmill study, I was quite aware of the fact that my capacity for exercise, so far as chest pain was concerned, was significantly better than it had been a year and a half ago. Likewise, as I watched my monitor, I was convinced that there had been a significant improvement to the circulation to my heart muscle as measured by the treadmill examination.

Having had a successful treadmill exam, I feel secure in continuing to accelerate my rehabilitation program with graduated physical exercise. I look forward to joining my friends on the golf course for a full eighteen holes. I expect to resume walking and carrying my golf bag.

Maintenance of the grounds and the grass on the greens around the lake has been a source of recreation in itself, as gardening is for many of my patients. I have always felt that physical activity that one can enjoy has an added benefit.

Never a high-wire rope walk again! I've had to answer to a lot of my friends, especially those who are patients, about my activities at the family retreat. I have to concede that the programs at a camp such as Eagle's Nest are planned for teenagers and young adults. I realize now that sixty-eight-year-olds should primarily be spectators rather than participants.

A number of years ago I was with a ski group in Switzerland and after enjoying the thrill of coming down one of the higher slopes in the Alps, I looked back and said, "Cliff Gaddy, I know you were not foolish enough to ski down from there!" It gave me such a sense of accomplishment that I never had the desire to do it again. I feel the same way about high-wire rope walks. Having achieved it once, and with the consequences that followed, I think I'll never have the desire to do it again.

I expect to be even more meticulous about my low-cholesterol, low-saturated-fatty-acid diet. I have added medication to further lower my total cholesterol, and hopefully to increase my high-density cholesterol so that I will have a much more favorable ratio between the two fractions.

There is always the question of resuming work. This will differ with each individual. Many who have bypass surgery will have already retired while others can resume the same hard physical work. I have been back to do desk work and a few consultations. I look forward to being back in the office on a regular basis.

I made rules long before the heart problem was manifest that I expect to follow. There were three requirements needed to keep coming to the office for regular daily work. They are as follows.

(1) There must be a definite need for my services. Many patients whose appointments were deferred during my absence have asked me to return as soon as possible. As long as work is scheduled two or three months in advance, I can assume there is a continuing need. My

associates in practice are as busy as they should be and certainly need help.

(2) Work must be satisfying. When I get up in the morning, I want to look forward to seeing patients. For all of these years I have preferred going to work more than anything else. I am sometimes asked, "If you were just beginning in life again, would you want to become a doctor?" I have always been able to answer definitely in the affirmative. There are many vocations that are interesting to me but none are nearly as appealing as my career in medicine has been. I would want to do the same thing—perhaps I could do it better.

(3) I must feel that I am fully competent to continue to do the best possible work for my patients. I would never want to work if my performance provided less than the best. It is most difficult for one to be objective about himself and his abilities. Many years ago I was in a position where it was my responsibility to determine whether a ninety-two-year-old physician was capable to remain on our hospital staff. Fortunately, it was not a problem because he was clearly competent, both mentally and physically, despite his age. Because I have successfully completed each and every recertification or self-assessment examination by the American Board of Internal Medicine for the past twenty-seven years, I feel qualified on this point. If there should ever be any indication of doubt, I hope one of my best friends will have the courage to tell me so. One of the greatest disasters in medicine is an incompetent physician still trying to work. Fortunately, organized medicine today is doing a much better job in protecting the public than in past years.

I expect to reduce my working hours and have more time for travel, for golf, and for other recreational activities. In other words, I am going to try to follow the routine that I have advocated for protecting the new grafts.

To make the eighth-week anniversary complete, it was the same day that Nez had the cast removed from her right arm. She is quite pleased with this, although there is still significant soreness in her wrist. She is able to do quite a bit more than she could do with the cast in place. I am quite happy to become less of a house husband. I must say that I was not much of one anyway.

I started swinging my 9-iron and doing a small amount of chipping about two weeks ago, and have gradually worked up to the 5-iron and 7-wood. I have successfully hit a few balls across the lake. There was no significant discomfort about the sternal incision. With my good treadmill test, I am now convinced that I am ready for my driver and the rest of my golf clubs. Who knows? I might find that my golf game has improved.

I recognize that I was fortunate in learning about the need for my cardiac surgery before my heart muscle was damaged. I am very grateful that my blockages were such that bypass grafts were readily performed with good results. I am also grateful that I have encountered no form of complication as a consequence of my donor-vein-graft surgery, the sternal incision, or the coronary artery surgery itself. I feel that I can definitely recommend that you should *never bypass a bypass operation*—that is, if you really need one!

Afterword

A year has now passed since my heart attack and surgery. Much has transpired during the course of this year in my personal life and in health care in general.

I've had the good fortune of having no further pain that could be attributed to my heart. Once my chest incision healed, I've had no limitation on my physical activity. At six-week and six-month intervals I underwent treadmill stress testing with very favorable results. The findings are much improved over those prior to surgery.

Discomfort in my neck and shoulders due to my old injury has continued to plague me. I have had much more intensive physical therapy and I am encouraged to take medications with mild analgesic properties for muscle relaxation. These have been helpful.

I have continued to work and have had the freedom to work primarily at my desired pace. However, this is never entirely possible when one is in clinical practice of medicine because the demands of patients are so varied and working hours are often longer than are scheduled or anticipated. Cooperative colleagues and excellent assistants have made this as favorable as possible.

I have become much more aware of the fallibility of physicians and recognize that we are human and make errors just like others. As Dr. Bernie Siegal says, M.D. does not stand for Medical Deity! You have probably recognized this several times in this sixty-eight-year-old cardiologist who used poor judgment in acting like a teenager while playing singles tennis, white-water canoeing over rapids, and especially traversing a high-wire rope walk designed for young adults.

The misinterpretations of a treadmill exercise test, generally a very accurate study, for me resulted in a near-fatal heart attack due to overexertion.

I have tried to deal more effectively with a familial cholesterol problem associated with a less-than-normal high-density cholesterol by taking medications designed to increase the HDL and lower the unfavorable fraction LDL. Failing to deal with this problem earlier likely led to the basic problem of cholesterol deposits in my coronary arteries.

I often think that if such errors in practice and management can occur in a trained cardiologist who has worked with thousands of patients for more than three decades, what chance does the average individual have, who does not have the benefit of such training?

During the course of this year, there have been efforts to revolutionize the methods of financing and delivering medical care. While it is obvious that change needs to be made, the question remains, "How can it be done?" We now have a new administration that proposes we have comprehensive care available for every citizen. While there is without doubt some waste, some inefficiency, and even some fraud in the American health delivery system, correction of these factors will not come close to covering the costs of the extended medical care suggested. Medicines are too expensive, but pharmaceutical companies will expect to operate at a profit and research and development will have to continue.

Protection against malpractice adds significantly to the cost of the health delivery system. But how much reform can we anticipate when those who are primarily responsible for legislation, namely lawyers, would have to bring about that change?

Because of rapidly advancing technology in medicine, whether coronary bypass surgery, percutaneous dilatation of arteries, or heart transplants, procedures are not likely to become cheaper. One could say the same thing about liver, lung, and other organ transplants, including the increasing demand for bone marrow transplants.

We must be willing to spend less on incurable, terminally ill patients, especially the very aged. We cannot promise the best possible care for every individual and anticipate doing this without an enormous growth in both bureaucracy and cost.

I have tried to emphasize the importance of good preventive medicine, especially as it applies to heart and blood vessel disease. The same must be done for cancer and the other leading causes of premature death. This is our only real hope for having healthier individuals at the least possible cost. If this book is successful in encouraging individuals to practice better health habits, my efforts will not have been in vain.

October 1993 *Clifford G. Gaddy, M.D.*

Appendix

Good Wishes from Eagle's Nest Camp

Rich Campbell, who was Director of the Eagle's Nest Camp during our weekend stay, had learned about my coronary bypass surgery by way of Steve. Since we were all packed to leave and I had given him a check for the fine services he and his staff had rendered, we departed without telling him that I was having discomfort in my chest. I was so favorably impressed and flattered by his letter of December 7, 1992, that I want to share it with you.

December 7, 1992

Dear Dr. Gaddy,

I hope this finds you resting quietly and recuperating quickly. We were shocked to learn of the complications that arose after you left. Our prayers were with you during that time.

Your energy, nerve, and vitality are an inspiration to us all. It is also reflected in your family. Everyone is simply charming. For that, you must be proud.

We at Eagle's Nest are happy to have been a part of your family reunion. Images of particular fondness of me are: our conversation the first night about golf, the mountains, etc.; Spite and Malice; and the campfire. Those images are still vivid, clear, and cherished.

I send prayers and thoughts to you for a healthy recovery, and I wish you and yours a warm, thoughtful, and spirited holiday season.

Godspeed,

Rich

I can't say enough about the favorable impression I had of Eagle's Nest Camp. On the Eagle's Nest Foundation letterhead is the following: "Experiential education for young people, promoting the natural world and the betterment of human character; chartered non-profit in 1945."

It is quite easy for me to see now why Steve wanted to have his three daughters there at camp during the last several years. Heather has been chosen to be a junior counselor during the 1993 season.

About the Author

Clifford Garland Gaddy, M. D., was born at Lake View, South Carolina, in 1924. After graduating from Lake View High School at the age of sixteen, he entered Wingate College and subsequently received his Bachelor of Science degree from Wake Forest University. He was inducted into the Army while at Wake Forest and spent one and one-half years in service during World War II. He was released from service to enter Bowman Gray School of Medicine of Wake Forest University where he graduated in 1947. He did a year of cardiovascular research in the Department of Physiology at Bowman Gray School of Medicine before entering his graduate medical studies at the University of Virginia Hospital in Charlottesville. There he did his internship, residency, and fellowship in Medicine before becoming an instructor in the Department of Medicine. In 1952 he entered the clinical practice of medicine in Danville, Virginia, where he has since practiced internal medicine and clinical cardiology.

Dr. Gaddy has served as president of the Memorial Hospital Medical Staff of Danville and as president of the Danville-Pittsylvania County Medical Society, and is a recipient of the Junior Chamber of Commerce Outstanding Young Citizen Award. He has served as president of the Danville Rotary Club, and has been honored as a Paul Harris Fellow. He has served as chairman of the board of deacons of the First Baptist Church of Danville, Virginia.

Dr. Gaddy is a member of the American Society of Internal Medicine and served on the board of directors of the Virginia State Society of Internal Medicine. He is a member of the Virginia State Medical Society and a member of the American Medical Association. He is certified by the American Board of Internal Medicine. He is a fellow of the American College of the Physicians and a member of the American College of Cardiology. He continues to practice medicine on a part-time basis in Danville, Virginia.

While in medical school, Dr. Gaddy married a nurse and long-time friend, Inez (Nez) Chapman. They now have six children and thirteen grandchildren. They reside at Westridge, Danville, Virginia.

♥